GREAT HAIR!

covers the basics for making your hair as beautiful
as it can be, with hints on . . .

PICKING A SALON

Learn how to investigate salons and pick a stylist
who will listen to *you*.

STYLING THE EASY WAY

Find out how to create salon-perfect styles that
only *look* like they took hours.

FINDING YOUR LOOK

Learn how to pick the perfect cut for your hair
type, face shape, and lifestyle.

And More!

GREAT HAIR!

Sallie Batson

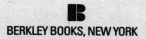

BERKLEY BOOKS, NEW YORK

GREAT HAIR!

A Berkley Book / published by arrangement with
the author

PRINTING HISTORY
Berkley edition / October 1995

For information address:
The Berkley Publishing Group, 200 Madison Avenue,
New York, New York 10016.

ISBN: 0-425-15022-4

BERKLEY®
Berkley Books are published by The Berkley Publishing Group,
200 Madison Avenue, New York, New York 10016.
BERKLEY and the "B" design
are trademarks belonging to the Berkley Publishing Corporation.

PRINTED IN THE UNITED STATES OF AMERICA

10 9 8 7 6 5 4 3 2

This book is joyfully dedicated . . .

. . . to my late parents, Davis Lipscombe and Irene Mc-Call Batson, who never failed to encourage my creative spirit; to the late Hal Waters, my professor and mentor, who taught me how to turn my talent into a craft; to all those editors along my way who insisted on excellence; to Linda Fine, who gave me my first pile of hairstyle photos to caption; to Stanley Harris, Phyllis Goldstein, and Mary Greenberg, who allowed me to edit *Hairdo* and *Hairstyle* all those years; to all the stylists and readers who give me so much to write about; and to Robert Bannard, who reminds me that, while I may know a lot about a lot of things, I don't know everything, and who makes me laugh.

Special Thanks:

Colin Lively of New York City, Cleveland, Ohio, and Palm Beach, Florida, my technical advisor

Frances London DuBose and the staff of London Hair, Charleston, South Carolina, and their models

Richard Peterson of New York, Cleveland, and Palm Beach

Robin Russo of New York

Donna J. Pollard of Cleveland, and her models

Lee and the staff at Ken Taranto Photography Services, New York, who salvaged the pictures *I* took

Intercoiffure America-Canada

The staff and students of Learning Institute of Beauty Sciences, New York City

My sisters Peggy Batson Ballard, Jan Davis Batson Childers, and Tally Batson Cobb

Mary Foster Conklin Ciaccio

Gloria Brown Gabin

Harry and Patricia Lapham

Adam Mars

Wu and Tony Palazolo

Lynette Sheldon

Hattie Wiener

MAKEUP STYLIST/New York
Samuelle Easton

MODELS/New York

Lisa Berkley	Marisabel Román
Elaine Bert	Robin Russo
Aileen Boyle	Stephanie Sfara
Ann Castillo	Lynette Sheldon
Ineta Chiliajaite	Gianna Skeete
Mary Foster Conklin	Kirsten Stendevad
Toyia Green	Nila Walker
Heather Jackson	Hattie Wiener

Tops worn in all photos taken by Jorge Ochoa are by French Rags, courtesy of Dominique Isbecque.

CONTENTS

GREAT HAIR!

1 HAIR'S LOOKING AT YOU, KIDS

We are known by our hair color or style: The Blonde Bombshell, The Beautiful Brunette, That Tall Red-Haired Lovely, The Girl with the Frizzy Brown Hair, The Long Ponytail. In fact, our hair is perhaps our most prominent identifying feature, even more than our skin color and body type are.

Even so, why all the fuss?

To begin with, there are approximately 140,000 hairs—an estimated 1,000 per square inch—on the average adult scalp. And some mornings, every one of these hairs seems to have a mind of its own.

Without the right cut, styling techniques, and products to control that willful growth atop our heads, we are setting ourselves up for one bad hair day after another.

WHY DO WE HAVE HAIR ON OUR HEADS?

Contrary to prevailing obsessions, the primary purpose of the hair on our heads is *not* to drive us nuts. Nor is its sole purpose to make us look a little bit different from the woman across the street. You can't even say that we have hair to make a fashion statement.

Hair grows out of our scalps to protect our heads from the elements. Period.

Remember how your mother insisted that you wear a hat every time you walked out the door in the wintertime? She was right. Massive amounts of body heat escape through our heads when we are without a protective covering.

And in the summer, our skulls would simmer in the sun without this natural chapeau.

Either way, you can imagine how rough it is for someone with no hair.

So that is why we have hair on our heads.

WHAT EXACTLY IS HAIR?

Hair, known formally as *pilus,* is a threadlike filament extending through the pores of the skin. It is 97 percent protein, with the remaining 3 percent composed of amino acids, minerals, and other trace elements.

We humans have some type of fuzz all over our bodies—except for our lips, the palms of our hands and the soles of our feet. In this book, the only hair we'll be discussing is on our heads.

A hair has three very distinct layers. On the outside is the *cuticle,* which is composed of flat, transparent, overlapping shingles that protect the inner part of the hair shaft. Should these cells become uneven or damaged, hair can lose its sheen or, in especially bad cases, result in split ends.

The second layer, or *cortex,* is made up of elongated cells growing end to end. They give the hair its flexibility and tensile strength. These cells contain the pigments that provide our hair with its natural color. Your hair turns gray when this pigmentation is depleted.

In the center is the *medulla*—two rows of cells that grow side-by-side along the shaft. This layer determines the width of the strand, as well as its strength and elasticity. This is what determines if the hair is fine or coarse.

For all intents and purposes, hair is dead. At least the part we *see* is. Only the *papilla* is alive. Every follicle grows from this bulblike node or root which is nourished by blood vessels that course through the scalp.

A hair follicle grows about one-half inch per month for two to six years, then it goes dormant for three to four months. During this rest period, the follicle is released by the papilla so that a new hair can begin to grow. In time, the original hair strand is pushed out by the new hair that has been slowly climbing its way through the skin.

Hair and scalp are lubricated by an oil, released by sebaceous glands through ducts that line the pores where the hair grows.

Bet you didn't know so much was going on up there.

When this growth-regrowth cycle is normal, the average life span of a healthy human hair is four years.

WHEN HAIR DOESN'T GROW RIGHT

A healthy person can expect to lose between eighty and one hundred hairs every day. This means that both the hair with its root and the scalp with its complex network of nerves and glands, are in proper working order.

However, if you come out with a whole handful of hair when you run your fingers through it, or if you see a lot of hair on your pillow, in your brush, or in the tub after washing it, you have a problem. This means too many of your roots are letting go, if not dying off, at the same time. The result can be devastating. If roots are dead, new hair growth is impossible.

On the other hand, if you're *not* shedding, you have trouble of a different nature. This means that your roots are not producing new hairs. New growth depends upon how much nourishment the papilla gets from the bloodstream and how clean your scalp is. New hair can't push its way through an oil-clogged scalp.

Either way, you need to do something. I'll go into more detail about chronic hair loss in a later chapter, but here are some immediate steps you can take to come to grips with less than perfect hair.

- Talk to your stylist. It could be that you've been doing something to damage your hair and scalp or that you are using the wrong hair care and styling products. Do you color your hair at home? Do you have a perm? Color *and* perm? It could be caused by any number of things. You may not be washing your hair correctly. We'll get into that later.
- See your dermatologist if you have persistent dandruff (dry, scaly scalp) or dermatitis (bumps and breaking out on your scalp or around your hairline).
- Also, take a look at your overall health. Have you been ill? Are you taking any medications? Have you been under a lot of stress?
- Do you work or live in an environment with lots of air pollution? Airborne grit and grime are extremely damaging to human hair.
- Take a close look at your diet. If it's high in oils and fats, especially red meats, fried foods and most nuts and nut products, you may be asking for trouble. Despite what you may think, a balanced, nutritious diet really is part of an effective haircare and styling routine.

BRUSH FIRST

Before you wash your hair, wrap your hairbrush in cheesecloth or gauze and run it through your hair. Work from scalp to ends. The fabric will absorb dirty oil residue, while the brushing loosens grit stuck to the hair shaft and scalp. You'll be amazed at how clean your hair will be!

WHAT KIND OF HAIR DO YOU HAVE?

Before you decide how you will wear your hair, you need to know a few things about it. Is it straight or curly? If it is curly, how curly is it? Thick or thin? Fine or coarse?

This is not always as simple as you might think.

My hair is very fine and, for the most part, thick. It is thin on top, thanks to a bad perm five or six years ago. It broke off at the scalp and never quite grew back to its original lush thickness.

To say that it's straight or curly is not so obvious. When I was a child, it was either cut short—in which case it was very straight—or permed—which meant it was very curly.

Once I grew old enough to protest this obligatory summer permanent-waving ritual, I started wearing my hair in a sleek, shoulder-length, pageboy bob. For this, my hair was all one length, blunt cut just below my chin line and curving across the back. Every night, I rolled it under on large, bristled rollers. For all I knew, it was as straight as a plumb line. Imagine my surprise years later when I had my hair cut in layers and found that it fell in soft, easy waves!

Fortunately for me, I've entrusted my hair to an absolutely brilliant hairstylist who knows what to do with it and makes sure I know how to handle it between visits. It's amazing how much easier it is for me to look good now that I know what I'm working with.

Hair's straightness or curliness depends on how it grows. When the root is positioned so that the follicle grows straight out of the scalp, the hair is *straight*. When the root is at an angle, so that the hair has to work its way out through the network of glandular ducts and nerves under the scalp, that hair is *curly*. The degree of the slant determines the amount of curl: the sharper the angle, the curlier the hair.

Other ways we characterize hair are to describe it as *fine* or *coarse* and *thick* or *thin*.

Simply put, *fine* hair strands are narrow; *coarse* hairs are fatter. This is determined by the thickness of the medulla. Fine hair looks great in blunt cuts, while coarser hair thrives when it's layered and feathered.

Finally, if you have *thick* hair, you have a lot of hair on your head. If it is *thin,* you have fewer strands of hair per square inch of scalp.

WHICH TYPE IS BEST?

So, which type is ideal?

Yours.

As long as you understand what your hair wants to do, you will always look your best. Straight hair wants to be straight; curly hair wants to curl. It's that simple.

When you fight with what your hair wants to do naturally, you will always lose. The only reason for you to have a bad hair day is that you have expected your hair to do something that it wasn't meant to do.

If you have any doubt as to what your hair type is, ask your stylist. If you don't ask, you'll keep on having hair that demands a lot of attention, and a lot of help.

2 HOW TO FIND THE RIGHT HAIRSTYLIST

A woman's search for the right hairstylist is almost as exacting—and every bit as personal—as her quest for the proper physician or a husband.

After all, your stylist is the person who determines whether your hair is your crowning glory or it gives Medusa a run for her money.

An ideal place to begin this search is with your friends, neighbors, co-workers . . . anyone you meet. If you like the way someone's hair is cut and styled, ask who did it.

Don't be afraid to talk to strangers. It is a great compliment to be asked who does your hair. Most women will be delighted to share their stylists' name with you. Just make sure that you get the salon's name and phone number. There may be more than one Ricardo or John in your community, and after all your sleuthing, you wouldn't want to go to the wrong person!

As traumatic as it can be to have a *bad* haircut, you can find solace in the knowledge that *hair grows back.* Unless you've ended up with a crew cut when you expected a chin-length bob, you only have to wait two to four months for your bad cut to grow out. It takes longer—about a year—to get over a bad perm or catastrophic color job, although an able stylist can help you with some interim relief. Or, you can cultivate a stunning wardrobe of hairpieces, hats, and scarves.

The best way to avoid such calamities is to talk things out with your stylist *before* he or she picks up a pair of scissors—before one strand is snipped.

STRATEGIES FOR A SUCCESSFUL SEARCH

Whether you are a newcomer to a community or just ready for a change in stylists, you can follow these leads:

- Head for the mall . . . or any other place where you will see a lot of people. Purpose of this trip is not to find a salon but instead, to spot people who have cuts and styles that you like. Approach them with a smile, introduce yourself (a great way to meet people if you are new to an area), and ask them who does their hair.
- Look in the Yellow Pages and local newspapers. Find ads that appeal to you, ones that show some style and imagination, not just a list of product names and services. Such ads indicate that the salon is a little bit more than your run-of-the-mill beauty shop. Then pay a visit to check it out for yourself.
- Call the beauty and fashion editor of the local newspaper and ask for her recommendations. She probably won't give you just one name—that wouldn't be particularly diplomatic, since hair salons advertise in her newspaper—but she should be able to supply you with the names and numbers of some reputable stylists.

Once you have compiled a list of possible salons, check them out. No matter what people have said about a shop, if every woman in every chair is a gray-haired grandma and you don't fit that picture, this may not be the right place for you. Likewise if you are a 35-year-old lawyer, and you see a lot of tattooed biker babes with nose rings and chunky cuts in neon colors, you might want to head for the next salon on your list.

- Go in for a manicure. What better way to spend a half hour or more in a shop without spending a lot of money? Nail polishing stations are almost always positioned prominently to give you a great vantage point. Besides, the manicurist might be a notorious gossip and willingly tell you who is the best stylist in the salon.

- If the salon does not offer nail service, simply ask to see its style books. Most shops, especially the chains and those affiliated with Intercoiffure America-Canada and the National Cosmetologists Association—professional societies for the beauty industry—train their operators in current styles and keep a photo scrapbook of these looks. This will give you a chance to get the feel of the work this salon does.

- You can also ask for a consultation. This is an appointment with either a stylist who has been recommended to you or someone the manager suggests, solely to discuss what can be done for you and your hair. You might want to schedule this appointment as soon after a cut as possible. This will give your future stylist an idea of what you have been happy with in the past. This is especially important if you are moving to a new community.

WHAT PRICE BEAUTY?

Is a stylist's price a valid gauge of his or her worth? Not exactly. There are a lot of exceptional stylists—especially in smaller cities and towns—who are quite moderate in their pricing.

A salon's price range will give you an idea of the type of service you can expect, though.

VALUE OR FAMILY PRICE SALONS
Price range: $7 to $10 per haircut; additional for other services.

Usually located in little strip malls, near popular grocery stores, or across the street from a larger mall, these shops prominently advertise their super-low haircut prices. This may be a bit misleading since pricing is rather à la carte. Customers pay for services individually, from the shampoo to the conditioner to the cut, comb-out, and blow-styling. By the time you're through, you could have gone to a full-service, mid-price salon and had a cut by a more experienced stylist for the same price.

Additionally, it is important for you, the client, to know that these seemingly low-price hair houses are usually staffed by newly licensed beauty school graduates. And, while beginning stylists can be very talented, you cannot expect to get the same sort of experienced service here as at a full-service, more upscale, salon.

BASIC MALL SALONS
Price range: $10 to $25 per cut, depending upon region. These are basic haircut houses. Most are chain salons

where customers can walk in without an appointment and get a hair cut. These are high-volume shops that cut a lot of hair. They usually have a book of pictures of the cuts their stylists are trained to do. If you see a picture that you like, chances are someone on staff has been trained to do it.

You're not necessarily going to get your worst cut, neither will you get your best hair*style*. You will find that these are highly functional salons noted for their convenience and moderate pricing.

LUXURY SALONS

Price range: $25 and up.

Usually in big cities, in affluent neighborhoods, or in up-scale malls, many of these salons offer so many services they are called "day spas". You will, no doubt, find a high-profile stylist—usually the owner—styling the hair of well-known, high-profile women. Even the lesser known operators in these temples of beauty have paid their dues and know their profession.

You can expect to receive top service for your hairstyling dollar in these salons. This means that your stylist will give you more chair time—time to talk about how you want to look and to learn exactly what you can expect from your hairstyle. Time spent on such communication is an essential part of developing your style . . . and it definitely makes you feel so taken care of that you want to go back.

WHAT DOES ALL THIS MEAN?

Buying a hairstyle is not at all the same as buying a blouse. You cannot try on several cuts and styles and then select the one that works best. Even if you look at pictures, you really won't be able to see how a cut will look until it is done.

Computer imaging, which allows the operator to position assorted styles and even colors over your Polaroid headshot, is a step in the right direction . . . but it is still only a step.

The only sure way to find the perfect stylist—and, in turn, the perfect style—is to keep talking.

3 HOW TO TALK
TO YOUR STYLIST

You can count on a good stylist to be a lot of things: Mindreader is not on the list.

Intuitive, yes; psychic, no.

If you are going to get the hairstyle of your dreams, you and your stylist must be in sync. You have to talk the same language, so that neither of you is surprised by the outcome.

If you have three hairs per square inch on your head, you cannot expect to look like Jane Seymour, with her lush, wavy tresses. The body-building products and styling techniques have not been invented to work this kind of magic.

Likewise, if you have super-curly locks, you will not be able to have that sleek pageboy bob unless you are willing to blow it out, set it on giant rollers, or straighten it chemically.

Now based in New York, Colin Lively owned salons in Cleveland, Ohio, for more than fifteen years. He comments, "I've spent many hours with crying clients who say, 'I didn't get what I asked for. This isn't what I said I wanted.' And I've spent equal hours with crying stylists who say, 'I gave her exactly what she told me she wanted.' It's as though they were speaking two different languages."

First of all, if both you and your hairstylist have unrealistic expectations about what one visit can do, you are bound to be disappointed. It takes at least three visits—a cut plus two trims—before you both will feel 100 percent satisfied with your hairstyle.

Since hair is part of fashion, and fashion is shaped by public personalities, you can communicate an easily identified image by using a celebrity name your stylist will recognize for her hair—Heather Locklear, Paula Zahn, Kathy Lee Gifford . . . Liza Minelli, Oprah Winfrey, Linda Evangelista.

Pictures make a great consultation tool. You can select possible looks from the salon's style book or clip pictures from magazines that appeal to you. Either way your stylist will appreciate knowing more about your taste.

Pictures are almost essential when talking about coloring your hair because color is so subjective. *You* may say "golden blond" thinking it will make you a shade that's honey kissed by the sun but end up as yellow as an Easter chicken. Or you may think that the red your colorist is describing will turn your mousy brown locks a glorious auburn when, in reality, it will make them closer to an *I Love Lucy* red.

There are a lot of variables to consider when sitting in that chair before a new hairdresser. Let's start with the hair on your head. It carries with it the results of all the haircuts, the perms, the colors . . . not to mention the shampoos and gels that you've put into it, the hours spent in hot rollers, and the months of drying time. The person who cuts and styles your hair needs to know about this, and more. That henna and chamomile rinse from the health food store may have given your hair highlights but it could cause hellish results when your stylist applies permanent waving solution. It's up to you to tell the truth.

- Do you have time, and are you willing, to spend more than 10 minutes a day styling your hair?
- *Can* you do what it takes to style your hair? Do you really know how to blow it dry? Can you use a curling iron or rollers?

THAT ALL-IMPORTANT FIRST IMPRESSION

If this is your first time with a stylist, make certain that the person who will be cutting, coloring, or curling your hair sees you with dry hair . . . and gets to inspect it. This doesn't always fit the program at those fast-paced hair cutting emporia that operate like assembly lines, escorting clients to be shampooed and *then* to the stylist's station.

Stand your ground, especially if you're having your hair cut. Wet hair appears to be longer and straighter than dry. Not even the most experienced stylist can calculate how much longer and straighter wet hair will be.

You also want to be wearing your typical weekday, workaday wardrobe and makeup when you meet a new hairdresser. This shows him or her how you dress most of the time. The result could be disastrous if you don't.

I had a neighbor who works for a very conservative Wall Street brokerage firm. For years, she wore her dark brown hair blunt cut one length at her shoulders, usually pulled back with a tortoiseshell headband or gathered to the nape of her neck by a simple barrette. Very simple; very safe; ultimately corporate.

Then her stylist moved away and she went to someone else—a talented stylist at a reputable top-line New York salon. Her first appointment was on a crisp Saturday morning in October, and she wore her ordinary weekend uniform—

jeans and a T-shirt, Doc Martens and a rather raunchy leather bomber's jacket. She told her new haircutter that she was bored with her bob and wanted something different. Then she settled back for him to work his magic.

She left the salon absolutely delighted by her exciting new 'do—cut to curve over one ear, with hair angled across the back so that it swung forward to the chin on the other side. The top was brushed across the crown and then forward so that it all but hid one eye. It also had shimmering ruby-red highlights.

She was the hit of the party Saturday night and won raves from her sister at Sunday brunch. However, on Monday morning, when she put on her austere, albeit chic, business suit with silk blouse, she realized that her trendy new look was not suited for her 9-to-5, Monday-through-Friday life. She quickly moved her 9 o'clock appointment to late afternoon and called the salon for emergency care. She ended up with a close-cropped cap style . . . and had the red highlights toned down considerably.

And she never went to that salon again.

WHAT YOUR STYLIST NEEDS TO KNOW

In addition to telling your stylist how short you want your hair cut or if you want it colored, you need to be up front about your physical well-being, your haircare and treatment history as well as your lifestyle.

- Are you pregnant? You should *never* have chemical processes, such as color, while you're pregnant since the chemicals in the dye get into your system . . . and your baby's.

- Are you taking any medications? Even birth control pills and antibiotics can affect chemical procedures such as color, permanent waving, or straightening.
- What is your lifestyle? If you are the mother of three preschoolers, you'll want a quick and easy style that can be dressed up for special occasions, not a look that demands daily attention.
- What treatments—color, perm, etc.—have you done or plan to do to your hair? Even if it was eight months ago, that home perm may influence how your hair accepts color now. Also, natural or herbal color and conditioning treatments can alter the cuticle and even the cortex of your hair. Your stylist needs to know this before proceeding with any chemical process or the results could be disastrous.

A WORD OF CAUTION

The more you change your hair from its natural state, the more you will have to do to it for it to look great. This is especially true if your hair has had a major color change.

Horror stories are legion. Just ask your stylist.

The worst of all possible problems can occur when a client who has bleached her hair blond goes in to a salon for conditioning and "color replacement therapy." Now her hair looks very natural. If she goes to a new stylist for a perm and this stylist, not knowing that there is bleach underneath, treats it like it is virgin, or untreated, hair, she will be in for a shock. Her hair is almost guaranteed to break off.

Color mishaps take a full year to grow out completely, and bad perms take even longer. However a trained stylist can help you with valuable remedies that will improve matters immeasurably.

Although hair nightmares seem to get a lot of publicity, most salon stories have happy endings.

4 PICK THE PERFECT LOOK FOR YOU

What makes a good hairstyle . . . and how can you tell if it'll be good for you?

Here are some questions you might want to ask when searching for a new look:

- Is it right for your hair type?

    Reread chapter 1 if you're still not sure if your hair is thick or thin, fine or coarse, etc. Remember: You want a cut and style that works *with* your hair.
- Is it suited to your face shape?

    Think of your hair as the frame for your portrait—your face. To look its best, your style should be shaped and proportioned to flatter your features.

    Slim down your round-as-the-moon face by directing hair forward to feather gently across your forehead, along your temples and about your cheeks. You will create the illusion of width by brushing hair loosely away from your long, narrow face. If your face is triangular, find a style which will widen the narrow portion of your face—layered through the crown to lend fullness about the temples; feathered at the baseline to bring a narrow chin into proportion with wide cheekbones. The angles of a square face, which appears to be as wide as it is long, will be softened by a cut that is layered along the hair's natural growth lines so that it lies easily about your face.

If you have any doubt as to what your facial shape is try this trick: Brush your hair away from your face and secure it with an elastic band or headband. Then stand in front of a well-lit mirror and trace the outline of your face onto the mirror with a grease pencil or a cake of soap. Then step back and decide, without question, if your face is round, square, oblong, oval . . . or even triangular.

• Is it the right proportion for your height and body build?

A hairstyle is part of your *total* look, not just from the neck up. A petite woman with delicate facial features might be dwarfed by too much hair, while a big, broad-shouldered gal will appear to be bigger and broader-shouldered with a short, close-cropped cut. This is not to say that a small woman cannot have long hair, or that a plus-size person won't look beautiful with short hair . . . provided it's in the proper proportion.

• Is it right for your lifestyle?

If you run or work out before work every morning, you certainly don't want a hairstyle that takes a lot of doing to look good. Likewise, if you work in a bank or a conservative law firm, you won't find a trendy cut, a fussy, upswept style, or a dramatic fashion color particularly appropriate.

THE CHOICE IS YOURS

Now is the time to pick a look you'll love. Here is a gallery of styles for your consideration.

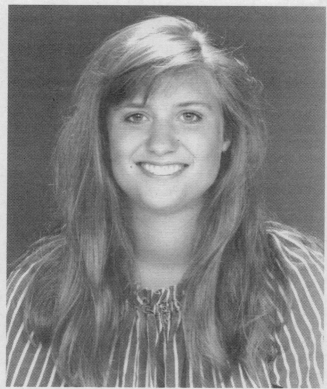

BEFORE

One could hardly call this haircut a style: Thick but fine hair falls loosely from a jagged side part. It can be worn down, like this; pulled back into a ponytail or braid; or tugged up on top of the head . . . and that's about it.

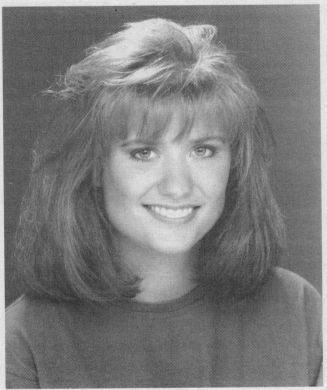

AFTER

You don't have to take off much length to create this sharp, sophisticated look. The base line is blunt cut at the shoulders, while underlayering starts in the crown, creating volume and distributing the hair's weight so that it swings with style. Bangs are cut straight across the temples and then featured to tickle the brow. This is one stunning blow-dry bob. It's long enough to pull into a French twist or curl on electric rollers for more dress-up occasions. HAIRSTYLE AND PHOTOS BY FRANCES LONDON DuBOSE.

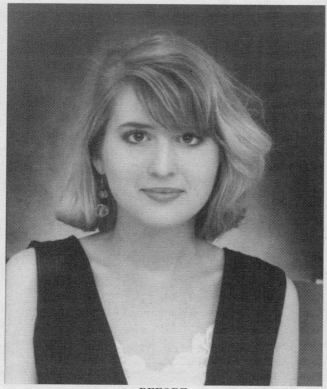

BEFORE

In dire need of an update, here's an eighties bob with thick bangs that angle across the brow from a high side part. The silhouette of this cut makes the face appear wide at the cheeks and chin line, and gives the look of a low forehead.

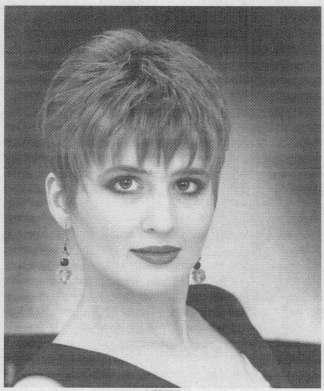

AFTER

Proportioned to enhance this model's delicate features and reveal her naturally oval face shape, hair is layered from the crown and clipped into soft wisps about the face. Vertical snips throughout the cut create height and texture. Highlights, painted through the layers of the original cut, add to the movement of this short, sassy style. Hair can be styled in minutes: Just fluff with your fingertips and pull it into place. If you're in a rush, blow dry as you finger-comb and shape your hair. HAIRSTYLE AND PHOTOS BY FRANCES LONDON DuBOSE.

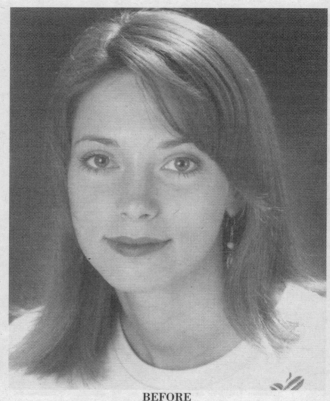

BEFORE

Fine, straight hair combed off a high side part accentuates the length of this model's narrow face. Because the hair has little body, it can only hang limply about the shoulders. Ends show the beginnings of splitting.

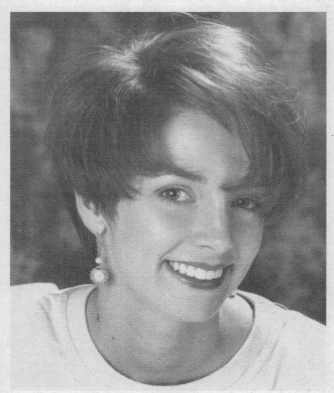

AFTER

Fullness in the crown teams with light feathering and diagonal bangs to lend softness and width to this model's somewhat angular face. All traces of split ends are removed, as hair is clipped to lie close to the nape. Underlayering adds volume to this cap-like silhouette. A snap to style with a blow dryer and vented brush, this cut is ideal for most straight or wavy hair types. Too much curl, be it permed or natural, would make it unmanageable. HAIRSTYLE AND PHOTOS BY FRANCES LONDON DuBOSE.

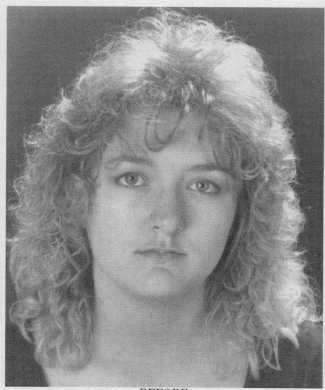

BEFORE

Overprocessing and sun damage render this curly bob lifeless, while the color is too far from the hair's natural color to flatter our model's skin tone. The overall length—at the collarbone—teams with the length of the bangs—close to the brow—to make her neck look short and her face wide.

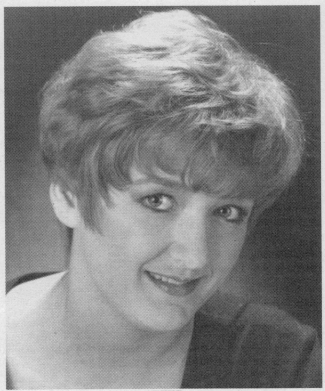

AFTER

Judicious cutting and serious conditioning restore this model's hair to health, while lowlights fill hair with hues that enhance her skin tone and eye color. Hair is layered to curve gracefully about the face, full through the top and gently tapered over the ears and across the nape. Bangs are full, swirling from the crown to brush the brow. The result is a soft, feminine frame for the face that works in perfect proportion to our model's features and body size. HAIRSTYLE AND PHOTOS BY FRANCES LONDON DuBOSE.

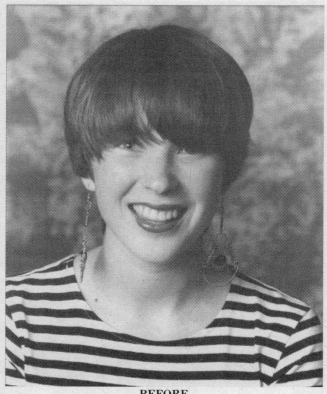

BEFORE

A short cap cut is perfect for thick, straight hair. The problem with this cut is that there's simply too much weight about the face. Aside from hiding our model's beautiful eyes, this down-sweep of hair emphasizes her somewhat sharp chin line.

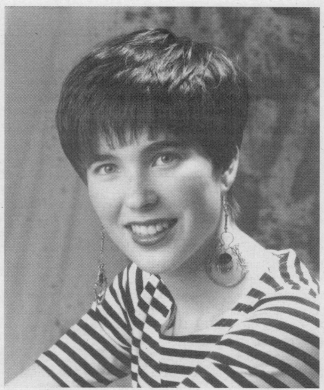

AFTER

What a quick way to lose some weight! Hair is clipped in short layers from the crown so that it fairly floats toward the face. Hair tapers to the temples and nape, with the base line curving sharply over the ears. This almost care-free cut is styled in minutes. Just add a bit of styling gel to towel-dried hair and comb into place. Fluff the crown with your fingertips or a vented brush as you blow it dry . . . or just leave it alone and let it dry in place. HAIRSTYLE AND PHOTOS BY FRANCES LONDON Du-BOSE.

SEAL SPLIT ENDS

A little olive oil will seal split ends. Apply lightly to dry hair, then wrap your head in a hot, damp towel. Cover with a plastic cap and let stand ten to fifteen minutes, until the towel cools. Then wash with a gentle shampoo, rinse and style as usual.

Of course, the only way to get rid of seriously damaged hair is to have a professional trim.

CONSIDER THE OPTIONS

I don't know about you, but I don't always want my hair to look the same way every day. After all, I don't *do* the same thing day in and day out. Sometimes I'm chained to my computer and telephone, and then there are days that are filled with meetings from dawn to dusk, not to mention weekends at the beach and nights on the town. Give me options. Options *I* can choose.

I feel the same way about my hairstyle. *I* want to be able to decide how I'm going to look. I don't relish being limited to just one look . . . and I certainly don't choose to be slave to my hair's whims. None of that "Well, Hair, what are you going to do today?" for me.

My favorite style starts with a blunt cut perimeter just below my chin line. It is layered just a little bit, to distribute its weight from the crown. (Because I have a *lot* of fine hair, it starts to look like I'm wearing a neck brace if it's too long or unlayered.) My bangs are long enough to brush forward, back or to either side, but not too long so I can't see where

I'm going. I can wear it loosely back at the temples with just part of the bangs flipped forward, or I can fluff everything forward to frame my face with irregular wisps. I can add height with a little teasing at the crown; gather the sides off my face with a barrette or combs, or I can set it on electric rollers for those dressier moments.

Now that's the kind of versatility I like.

CUT AND COLOR
Hair is cut straight at the base, even with the jaw line and across the nape. Layering follows the hair's natural growth pattern from the crown to create movement throughout the cut. Gold and copper highlights are painted through the layers of the cut, radiating from the face in a light, lively halo.

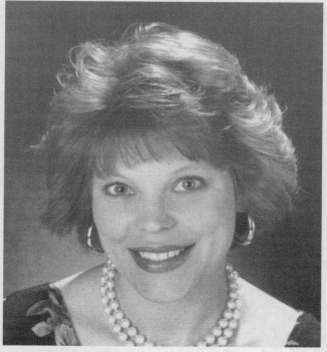

STYLING OPTIONS
For easy, everyday styling, simply apply a bit of spray gel—or use a light, leave-in conditioner—and lift with a vented brush as you blow it dry. Fluff the crown with your fingertips and pull a soft fringe across your forehead.

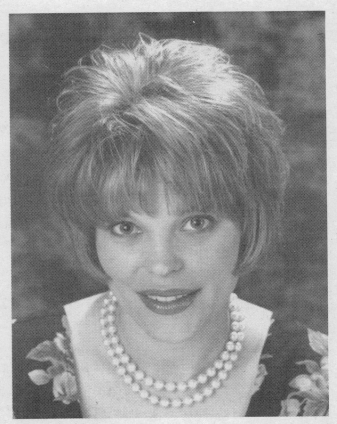

Create a softly rounded silhouette for this dressier style. Dab strong-hold gel at the roots and lift hair in sections with a circular brush. Direct hot air toward the roots as you curl it under and around the brush. Let each roll cool before releasing. Comb curls forward on the sides and shape thick bangs across the forehead. HAIRSTYLES AND PHOTOS BY FRANCES LONDON DuBOSE.

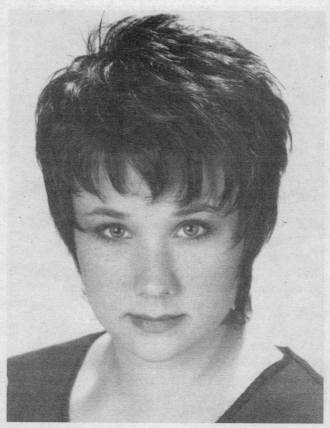

SUPER SHAG
It's fresh. It's feminine. It's a look that needs no special products or skill to style. It's the Shag . . . updated for the nineties.
Following its natural growth lines, hair is layered in easy spikes
about the face, with the back tapering close to the head. Run
your fingertips through gelled hair and pull forward to the
cheeks and across the forehead. Comb close to the neck in

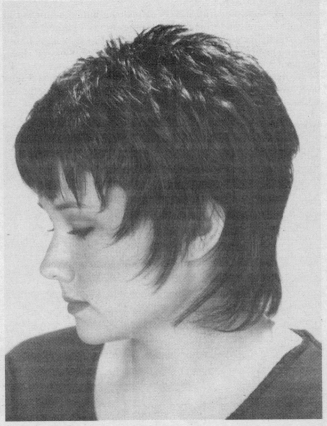

back, easing sides to the front. Let dry naturally and then run your fingertips through the top to loosen the line of the hair. This is a style suited to almost every hair type except very curly. HAIRSTYLE AND PHOTOS BY FRANCES LONDON Du-BOSE.

CUT AND COLOR

Long and thick, naturally curly or permed hair is blunt cut at
the bottom and underlayered to distribute its weight throughout. Highlights and lowlights intermingle through light blond
hair to accentuate the movement of the curl. For casual days,
just scrunch the curl with your fingertips as you blow dry. To
create these dramatic, dressy looks, dry hair completely. Spritz
each section with spray and make stand-up pincurls all over
the head, twisting each section as you roll the hair.

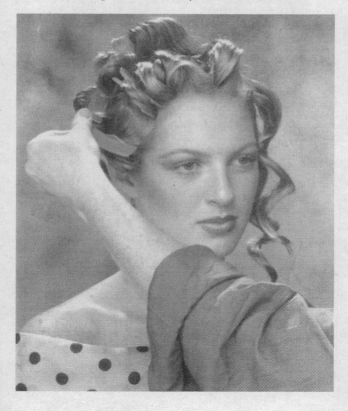

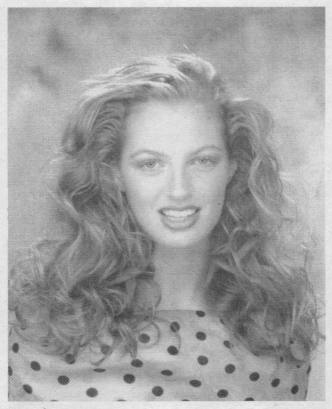

STYLING OPTIONS

To increase the fullness of this exquisite style, just lean forward so that your hair falls across your face and tease it lightly with your fingertips. Add a light spritz of spray if you need it because of the weather or because your hair is very fine. Then flip hair back and brush into place. Move bangs to one side and lift hair away from the temples, then let curls cascade gracefully about your shoulders.

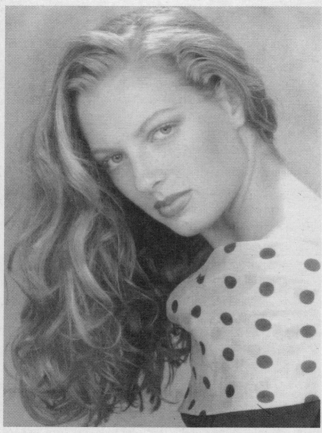

Swing hair seductively to one side for a sexy alternative style. Make a high side part and then brush hair across the back and secure with hairpins. Bangs move freely to tickle the brow. Just watch how the color dances with the curl! HAIRSTYLE BY STEPHANI McCRARY FOR LONDON HAIR. PHOTOS BY FRANCES LONDON DuBOSE.

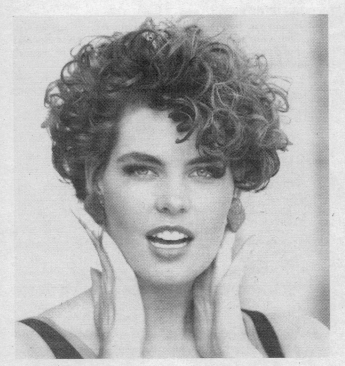

PARTY CURLS

Here is a sophisticated curly look that's just right for permed or naturally curly locks. Hair is layered all over, with fullness left through the crown. Sides and back are clipped close to the head. Golden highlights radiate from the hairline, defining the movement of both cut and curl. Roll gelled hair in random pin-curls—some stand-up and some traditional. Dry with diffused air or under lamps. Let cool before removing clips, then comb with your fingers. Move hair back at one temple, then fluff the other forward just a bit on the other side. Free curls so that they tumble loosely forward over one brow. HAIRSTYLE AND PHOTO BY FRANCES LONDON DuBOSE.

ONE BASIC CUT . . .

The baseline—or bottom perimeter—is cut straight across the back. Bangs are combed forward and cut straight across the brow. Following its natural growth patterns, hair is layered from underneath to distribute weight.

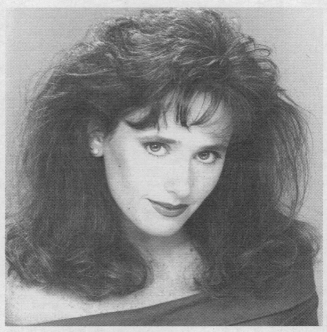

. . . TWO DIFFERENT STYLES

Coarse hair with a bit of natural curl and a lot of body lies just below the shoulders for a sophisticated, grown-up style. Layering through the crown adds lift. Bangs are slashed to fall forward in irregular curls. Comb gel through damp hair and blow dry, working hair off the face at the temples and curling loosely upward at the ends. Light teasing through the top will increase height.

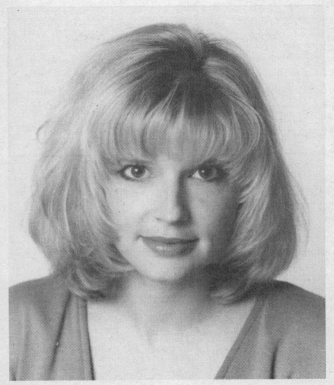

Fine, straight, shoulder-length hair looks sensational in this simple version of our basic bob. Long layers are angled around the face, making this a super style for round or square faces. Full bangs are combed forward from a short center part, while underlayers through the back enhance hair's volume beneath the satin-smooth silhouette. Gold and copper tones are brushed throughout the hair to define the movement of the cut. Blow gelled hair dry over a vented brush, then finish with a curved brush when styling the sides. HAIRSTYLES AND PHOTOS BY FRANCES LONDON DuBOSE.

EMERGENCY MEASURE

No time to wash? Give yourself a dry shampoo. Sprinkle cornstarch or baby powder *lightly* onto your hair and then brush it out. For best results, cover your brush with several layers of cheesecloth—or slip your brush into a cotton sock—to pick up dirt.

5 COLOR AND CURLS

The two most dramatic ways to change the appearance of our hair is to alter its color and to give it some curl.

Ideally, either process should only be done by professionals.

Realistically, it isn't. The hair and beauty industry estimates that eighty percent of American women, at one time or another, color their hair. I don't know the exact figure, but I suspect the percentage is also high for home perms.

Products manufactured and sold for home use are not inferior, but: 1. stylists are trained to look for damage an unskilled eye may miss; and 2. it is physically impossible to properly roll or apply color to the back of one's own head. A professional colorist also knows how to blend tints and tones and brush them through the layers of your locks to create highlights and lowlights that appear amazingly natural.

SO, WHAT ABOUT COLOR?

I don't know about you, but during my teens, everyone I knew experimented with everything from comb-in bleaches to lemon juice or hydrogen peroxide—combed throughout the hair and followed by a day at the beach—to put some zip

45

into our hair. (There may have been an element of wanting to irritate our parents, too, but that's another book.) Aside from making it feel like straw, I never managed to do more than turn my hair a ghastly, eerie green by swimming in a chlorinated pool and then sitting in the sun without washing it out. This required intensive hot oil treatments to repair the damage before I could return to school come fall. My best friend, Betsy, who had dark brown hair, always got sensational copper highlights. Regardless of the results, this is *not* the way to color your hair.

Hair starts looking dull and drab long before it turns gray. By our late teens or early twenties, it has lost most of its secondary tones, those shimmering highlights of our childhood. That in itself is enough to drive many women to reach for the bleach and toner years before it's time to cover any gray.

Such a pre-gray color change is called "fashion color." Artfully applied, color can accent the architecture or line of your cut. If your hair is light, you may want to brighten the prevailing gold or silver tone. And if your hair is dark and you want enhancement rather than change, you might elect to add gold or red highlights.

Hair color is a rather subjective, and consequently confusing, matter. That's why I interviewed an expert in the field, Colin Lively who's based at New York's Elizabeth Arden Salon. Rather than dividing hair into blond, red or brunette, he makes hair color very simple to understand, separating it into two very specific categories: light or dark.

"After all, blond can be pale gold, almost white or the color of an Easter chicken, and brown hair can range from a mousey tan to rich mahogany," he explains. "Light is light and dark is dark. You can't get subjective about that."

Hair is not just one color naturally. The most beautiful hair is alive with a multitude of complementary tones moving through it. That's the way it looks best in nature. Even if your hair appears to be dark brown, you will find an assortment of black, red, and even gold strands intermingled all over your head. It's just the primary color that's dark brown.

If you insist upon doing your own color, buy a frosting kit and *follow the directions to the letter.* If your hair is dark and you want a change, get that frosting kit and, instead of bleach, use a permanent hair tint that will give you the red or gold tones you desire. You certainly don't want to have that one-color-all-over look produced by ordinary bleach-and-toner home hair color kits. It's so unnatural . . . and unlovely.

RINSE AWAY RESIDUES

To remove hair spray buildup from blond and light-colored hair, mix ½ cup lemon juice concentrate with 2 to 3 cups tepid water. If your hair is dark, mix ¼ cup apple cider vinegar in 2 to 3 cups water. Add 1 teaspoon oil of cloves.

Pour through your hair and leave on for ten minutes or longer. Rinse with warm water for two minutes.

SO MANY COLORS IN THE RAINBOW!

Just look at the array of hair coloring products filling the shelves at your corner drugstore or on display at your favorite hair salon. The spectrum is spectacular.

Who cares how many color choices you have? You just

want to make the right choice. So, how do you decide what you're going to use, either on your own or at the salon? Look into your eyes. Eye color, far more powerfully than skin tone or prevailing hair color, is the deciding factor in choosing a flattering color.

Here are some guidelines, built on Colin's years as a stylist and colorist:

- *Blue eyes:* You can choose any color that strikes your fancy—from platinum blond to blue-black or anything in between.
- *Green eyes:* You have *almost* as much latitude as your blue-eyed peers. Just steer clear of the extreme hair shades—very pale, especially ash tones, or very dark.
- *Hazel eyes:* You'll find a mixture of warm tones blended with ash in hazel eyes. Because of this mix you'll want to keep your hair color neutral. Stay in the middle of the color spectrum—for instance, dark honey or dark ash blond; rich copper-red; light, caramel brown.
- *Light brown eyes:* The most prevalent combination is light brown eyes with medium to dark brown hair. You might want to add warm highlights to the basic color—especially around your face—to give your hair a lift.
- *Brown to dark brown eyes:* You'll look best with dark hair. This might be a dark auburn, with spicy ginger highlights, or a mahogany. Which shade or tone you select depends on whether or not you have flecks of gold in your eyes or not. If you have that golden glint, go for the red tones to enhance that inner warmth.

FOR EASY CLEANUP

If you insist on coloring your hair at home, apply a bit of petroleum jelly around your hairline to keep the dye from discoloring your skin.

THE COLOR COMMITMENT

Before you color your hair you must decide how much you are willing to commit to the coloring process and to maintaining this color. This is not a decision to make lightly. A lot of work goes into keeping those golden locks gold.

The three basic types of hair color products vary in how long they last:

• *Permanent color* is used to cover hair that is fifty percent gray or to provide a serious, marked color change. Roots must be retouched every four to six weeks, depending upon hair color and how fast your hair grows. It takes a deft hand to apply the color only to the virgin regrowth. If you let color stay more than three to five minutes on previously colored hair you may well cause serious damage to your tresses. In any case, you'll end up with hair that doesn't match from one end to the other—the newly colored hair will have one tone, the previously colored hair another. Repeated application of permanent colors can also produce bad results. Nonetheless, if you show respect for the condition of your hair, shampoo-in permanent colors are not only simple to apply, but they can be very safe to use.

- *Demipermanent color* covers moderate graying and provides life to dull, listless hair. These products shampoo in and last from six to eight weeks. You can create dazzling highlights with bright or contrasting colors because the light, gray hair provides a different base for the color than your darker, untreated hair does.
- *Semipermanent color,* like the demipermanent, covers gray and adds zip to drab hair, only it washes out in six to eight shampoos. This is a great way to try a new, even daring, hair color without risk. If you don't like the way a color looks, just keep washing until you're back to where you started!

Just follow the manufacturer's directions to the letter and you won't go wrong.

Sometimes these single-process color techniques are not enough. If you want to make your hair lighter than its natural color, you must prepare it, much like an artist readies a canvas by painting it with a layer of gesso or white paint. First you must strip the pigment from your hair and then replace it with the color or colors of your choice.

And in three or four weeks, you'll need to repeat the process on the new growth. You know what *that* looks like. Roots!

These touch-ups are a complicated process because you're dealing with two kinds of hair—treated and untreated, both on the same strand—and each must be dealt with differently. You will need to strip and tone the virgin growth without letting the bleach run into the previously colored hair. Then, for the last three to five minutes of the processing time, you work it through to the ends.

This alone should point you in the direction of a professional colorist. Root upkeep is a complicated process that, if not done correctly, can cause dryness and breakage. It can also leave you with as many rings as a tree trunk, one for every time you touch up your color. If you still want to do it yourself, I suggest at least getting a friend to help apply color products—especially in back. There's no way you can reach that area of your own head.

Don't get me wrong. Coloring can do great things for your hair. In addition to adding exciting dimension and movement to the color of your hair, it can add volume to fine hair. Also, today's home hair coloring products are far safer, and produce much more reliable results, than their predecessors. But in the long run, considering the root upkeep and the risks involved, coloring is a job best left to the professionals.

Once your hair has been colored, you must handle it with care. Never, ever, brush wet hair, and always, always, use low temperature if you blow it dry. Use steam curlers rather than older types of hot rollers and curling irons, and, if you're perming your hair, make sure your stylist uses one formulated for colored and treated hair. You'll also want to invest in shampoos, conditioners, and styling products made for colored and treated hair. It's worth the investment.

HENNA ALERT

Henna may be "natural" but it is not without its hazards. Don't use henna on hair that has been permed or colored and don't perm or color hair that's been dyed with henna. You could end up with a mess! Hair could break; color could be uneven; the perm might not take.

A MATTER OF CURL

Like coloring your hair, permanent waving changes the texture of your hair by saturating the hair shaft with chemicals.

And also like hair color, too much of a good thing can produce horrendous results. We all have seen hair that's as fuzzy as a Brillo pad after Thanksgiving dinner. Chances are this dry, damaged look is the result of too many perms, the wrong perm for the woman's hair type, or even bad rolling.

Today's perms are not like those foul-smelling solutions of the past. They are either almost odorless or more pleasantly scented to mask the caustic smell of the chemicals. Another improvement: They're designed to stop working after a specified amount of time. They also come in varying strengths and formulations—for hair that has never been colored or permed, for previously permed hair, and for colored hair.

It's important that you use the right product for your hair type and condition. Hair that has been chemically treated (previously permed or colored) will break off if you use a product formulated for virgin hair (hair that has never been chemically treated). Likewise, a perm formulated for previously treated hair is not strong enough to work on virgin hair. Initially, you might get *some* curl, but it won't last through two or three washings.

If you still need to be convinced that perming is not a do-it-yourself project, consider this: It is *physically impossible* to properly roll the hair on the back of your own head . . . unless you're a contortionist. The operative word here is "properly." When rolling hair for a perm, you must take care not to pull hair against its root or twist the strand as you coil it around the rod, because the chemicals that make the wave permanent swell the layers of the hair shaft and make it vulnerable to damage.

Hair should be divided evenly into sections. Each section is then wrapped with an end paper and rolled around the appropriate-sized rod. The trick is to make that roll without pulling hair back against the roots. Any tension at the root will weaken the hair shaft and foster breakage.

If you decide to perm at home anyway, make it a party. Enroll a friend to roll your hair and you return the favor and roll hers. At least you're more likely to get your hair rolled properly.

The best advice, again, is to leave perming to the professionals.

IT'S A MATTER OF TIME

Hair should not be colored and permed at the same time. Color first, then perm a week to ten days later, but not much longer.

If you wait too long between processes, you'll be dealing with two different types of hair—virgin regrowth and treated. And that can be a major problem.

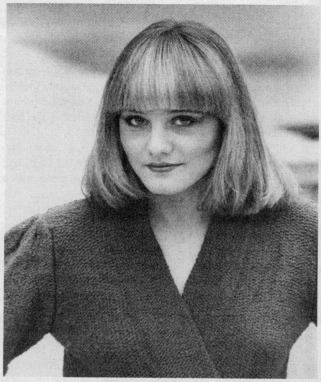

Natural-looking hair is not all one color. That's why this shimmering blend of highlights and lowlights looks so sensational. Thick, straight hair has been blunt cut at shoulder length, with long bangs combed forward from a short center part and clipped across the brow line from temple to temple. A rainbow of golden tones—from pale yellow to golden brown—are painted throughout, transforming light hair that's neither dark blond nor light brown into a vibrant study of movement and color. HAIRSTYLE AND PHOTO BY FRANCES LONDON DuBOSE.

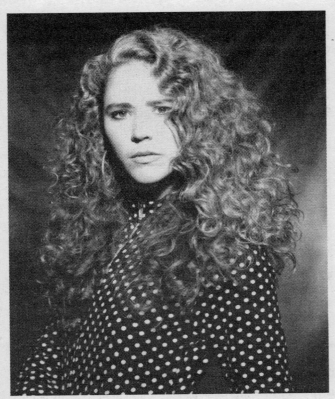

Color and curl cascade together in this long, flowing look that is styled by scrunching gelled curls into place with your fingertips as you blow hair dry. Large, medium, and small rods are used to roll hair for this natural-looking perm. Caramel highlights drip through the curl, creating warmth throughout the depth of this style. Hair is made lighter about the face to create both openness and warmth. Just remember: Color and permanent waving *cannot* be done on the same day. HAIRSTYLE AND PHOTO BY FRANCES LONDON DuBOSE.

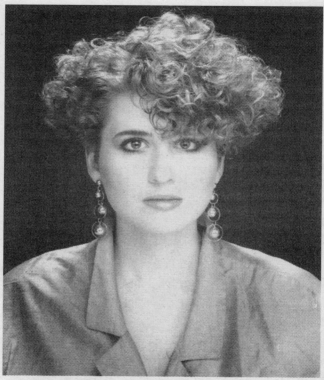

Give fine hair a lift, while making it a snap to style, by adding curl to a well-shaped cut. Hair is left full through the crown, with baseline cut close to the head. The lively variety of curls is created by rolling with rods of varying sizes—a small rod next to a medium rod—throughout the crown. To style, lift hair with your fingertips or a pick to free curls through the crown. Pull bangs forward and across one brow. Width created across the crown and at the temples makes this sophisticated style especially chic for the woman with a long, narrow face. HAIRSTYLE AND PHOTO BY FRANCES LONDON DuBOSE.

COLORFUL IDEAS

- Add a couple tablespoons of beet juice to your final rinse to give your hair rich, red highlights. Dark hair takes on lush jewel tones, while lighter hair gets a strawberry hue.
- Chamomile tea gives golden highlights to blond hair. So does a brew of marigold leaves, lemon juice, orris root, and elder flowers.
- Add $1/2$ cup strong coffee to your final rinse to give stunning mahogany highlights to brown or brunette hair.

6 HOW TO WASH YOUR HAIR

You just think you know how to wash your hair. What's not to know? You just rub some shampoo and water into your hair until it bubbles, and then you rinse it out. You've done it for years.

But that's not all you need to know.

You've got to know what kind of shampoo to use, and which conditioners and styling products work best for your hair. If you color or perm your hair, you have even more to consider.

Then there's the matter of technique. You can't just pick up a bottle of shampoo and squirt a blob on top of your head. You are about to learn the science of hair-washing.

START OUT WITH A GREAT SHAMPOO

You do not have to buy the most expensive, most popular, or even the newest product on the market. The first two ingredients of any commercially prepared hair-washing substance are water and a detergent—most often tea laurel sulfate, sodium laurel sulfate, sodium stearate, or some variation thereof. This is what makes the suds.

Except for preservatives and stabilizers, all the other ingredients are the bells and whistles that give the beauty business its mystique.

PICK THE RIGHT PRODUCTS

- Dry hair demands shampoos and conditioners rich in emollients; use alcohol-free gels, mousses, and styling products.
- For overprocessed, damaged hair, use a shampoo with a low pH, protein conditioners, and weekly warm-oil treatments.
- Thin hair needs a protein shampoo and conditioner and styling products with body-building ingredients such as balsam and resin.
- For oily hair, use alcohol-free, pH-neutral shampoos, detanglers, and styling products. Condition hair weekly.

These stabilizers and preservatives do nothing to clean our hair. In this latter category are sequestering agents, such as ethylenediamine tetraacetic acid (EDTA), which make the water soft to remove film and make the hair shinier. These ingredients prevent physical or chemical changes affecting color, texture, appearance, and even the flavor or scent of a product.

Other additives prolong the shelf life and marketability of the concoction. Scents, coloring, and emollients make it different from all the other shampoos on the shelf.

Finishing ingredients, such as lanolin, mineral oil, and wheat germ oil, make hair shiny. Humectants, such as honey, glycerin, and sorbitol, increase the hair's ability to absorb water, making it less brittle and more pliable.

Have no fear if you see some form of alcohol, hydrochloric acid, or some other ominous-sounding potions you vaguely remember from Chemistry 101 on the list. The alcohol in shampoos isn't the same as rubbing alcohol or what you find in nail polish removers. Cetyl and stearyl alcohol are opacifying agents—fatty alcohols distilled from sperm whale oil—that give shampoos, conditioners, and other hair- and skin-care lotions a creamy, opaque appearance.

You may find such acids—hydrochloric, oleic, citric, and others—toward the bottom of the ingredients roster and, consequently, having the least amounts in the formula. Used as preservatives and foam inhibitors, these additives help to restore your hair's acid mantle.

Read your labels to determine how much of these ingredients are in a product. If they are too high on the list, that product may be too harsh for your hair and scalp.

I won't launch into a rambling explanation—I'm sure I've already told you more than you ever wanted to know about hair care products in the first place—but I do want to stress that, if your hair is to be healthy, it should have a slightly acidic pH factor. This serves as a protective shield all the way through the hair shaft.

Herbal extracts and concentrates, such as white nettle, mistletoe, ivy, and chamomile, as well as aloe vera gel and avocado and jojoba oil, are often added to give you a sense that you're doing something natural (translation: healthy) for your hair and scalp.

Guess what? You are. White nettle is known to soften hair and add shine. It also stimulates hair growth. So will basil oil, mistletoe, and ivy. Avocado and jojoba oils in a shampoo have conditioning properties for both hair and scalp, while chamomile brightens light hair color. In highly concentrated form, it even turns dull hair bright golden blond. (I'll share some more natural hair coloring in chapter 5.)

A few more words about shampoo:

- When buying a new shampoo (or a conditioning or hair-styling product) resist the temptation to get the jumbo-gi-ant-economy size. How do you know if it'll deliver on its advertised promises? Instead, buy only enough to give the product a fair trial. A week's worth should do it.
- The amount of suds a shampoo makes has nothing to do with its ability to clean your hair. In fact, high-sudsing shampoos are often difficult to rinse completely from your hair. (Another bit of information about suds: The dirtier your hair, the fewer suds your shampoo—whatever brand—will produce.)
- Never dilute your shampoo unless the instructions give you the go-ahead. You'll never get enough detergent action to clean your hair if you do.
- If you're not a baby, don't use baby shampoo. A grown-up's body chemistry is not the same as a child's. Those gentle, tear-free shampoos aren't strong enough to clean an adult's hair and scalp.

AFTER YOU SHAMPOO

After you've rinsed all the suds out of your hair, you're ready to finish the process with something that will take out tangles and repair damage done by such things as bleaches and dyes, heat, cold, and air conditioning, not to mention aging.

Most conditioning products are applied to wet hair after

washing. Traditionally, they are rinsed out after three or four minutes—longer if you're using a deep conditioner or if your hair is especially damaged. However, many newer conditioners can be left in the hair for added body and protection.

While a cream rinse is relatively liquid, a conditioner is thicker, like a lotion. Spray-on conditioners are almost waterlike. Experiment with various products to see what works best for your hair type and style. Basic ingredients will vary only slightly. Differences will be found in such additives as color and scent. Manufacturers describe the properties of their products in glowing terms, so it is up to you to determine what you need and which brand or product you prefer.

Here's how conditioners work: Water softens the hair, making it more receptive to the humectants, finishing agents, and emulsions in the product. Additives may include protective sunscreens, color enhancers, and even protein—such as an egg or hydrolyzed animal protein—which bond with the hair shaft for added body and manageability.

Humectants, such as glycerin, urea, sorbitol, and propylene glycol, bring moisture into the hair and help to keep it from evaporating once on the hair. As a result, hair remains soft.

Finishing agents, such as balsam, quassia, acacia, or isopropyl myristate, leave a film on the hair that makes it feel soft and look shiny.

Most oils form emulsions with water. In conditioners, this might be lanolin, sterols, alcohols, spermaceti, glycerin, glyceryl monostearate, even olive oil and mineral oil. Emulsifiers coat the hair shaft and increase body.

- For best results, use the same brand of shampoo and conditioner. These products are made to work together.

- Shampoo-plus-conditioner products are not for all hair types. If you have doubts, ask your stylist if they're for you.
- Unless the directions suggest leaving a conditioner in your hair, take care that you rinse it from your hair. If you don't, it will weigh your hair down. (Keep reading. I'll tell you more about washing and rinsing techniques.)
- If you have colored, permed, straightened, or otherwise chemically treated your hair, request a consultation with your stylist to determine exactly what products you should use.
- If you still have any doubts about what products you should be using, ask your stylist to suggest conditioning products for your hair type, texture, and style. Why spend money on something you may not need?

IN GREAT CONDITION

Condition fine hair *before* washing rather than after. You'll be amazed at how much more body your hair will have.

THE RIGHT TECHNIQUE

Once you've chosen the right shampoo and conditioner, you're ready to wash your hair. Whether you wash it every day or every two or three, or whether you choose to hop into the shower or lean over a sink, you'll follow the same procedure.

Step 1: Brush your dry hair thoroughly to loosen dirt and grime; comb out any tangles. *(THIS* is the only time you might think of brushing those 100 strokes Grandma preached about.)

Step 2: Saturate your hair with warm to hot (but not scalding) water.

Step 3: Squirt or pour a small amount of shampoo—a dollop about the size of a quarter for short to medium-length hair; the size of a silver-dollar for long or thick hair—into the palm of your hand. Rub your hands together.

Step 4: Rub shampoo into your hair, starting with the hairline in front and continuing through the ends.

Step 5: Work up a lather, using the pads of your fingertips. Starting at the front hairline, make small circles, first at the top, then the temples. Add a little water if necessary. Continue making these little circles in the scalp, working across the crown and across the back.

Step 6: Make zigzag movements across the crown of your head and then up and down across the back, making certain that the ends of your hair are covered with lather.

Step 7: Slide your open hands through your hair to remove most of the excess suds.

Step 8: Starting at the front hairline, rinse shampoo from hair with warm to tepid water. Continue running water through your hair until the water runs clear, from three to five minutes.

Step 9: Repeat this process if your hair was especially dirty or if you use a lot of hairspray or styling gel. If you have short hair or if you wash your hair daily, one lathering is sufficient.

Step 10: Pour a small amount of conditioner into palm of your hand. Rub your hands together.

Step 11: Start rubbing conditioner into the ends of your hair. Work your way up the hair shaft to the roots.

Step 12: Gently comb conditioner through your hair using

a comb with wide, rounded teeth. This distributes the conditioner through your hair while helping to remove tangles.

Step 13: After three to five minutes, or according to directions, run warm to cool water through hair to rinse out conditioner. Finish with a blast of cold water to seal conditioners into the hair shaft. This leaves hair extra shiny.

Step 14: Blot excess water from your hair with a thick terry towel. Then lift hair in sections and gently rub dry with a towel, taking care that you don't grind the delicate strands into the cloth.

Step 15: Starting with the ends, comb hair with your wide-tooth comb to remove any new tangles.

Step 16: Style and dry hair as desired.

The entire washing and rinsing process can take from five to twenty minutes, depending upon the length and condition of your hair.

THE PERFECT FINISH

No need to spend big bucks for special "sealing" or "finishing" products for your hair. Add 1 cup cider vinegar to 1 gallon warm water and pour it through your hair as a final rinse. This solution protects your hair shaft by restoring its natural acid mantle.

EVERY DAY ... OR ONCE A WEEK?

How often should you wash your hair? That's for you to decide. You might want to wash your hair every day:

—If your hair is short and straight.

—If you use a lot of styling products—gels, sprays and the like. In this case, you'll want to use a clarifying treatment such as a vinegar–water rinse once a week to dissolve the residue that's stuck to your hair shaft.

—When you've been playing tennis, mowing the lawn or engaged in some other activity that has you in a sweat.

—If you smoke or if you've spent any time in smoke-filled rooms.

—If you work or live in an area where the atmosphere is filled with airborne pollutants.

—When you get caught in the rain . . . or go walking in the snow.

You may want to wash your hair every *other* day:

—If your hair is oily. Daily washing merely signals your sebaceous glands to produce more oil.

—If your hair is coarse and dry—and if you're using products specifically for coarse and dry hair, you may wait even longer to wash.

—If your hair is very long and/or thick, taking a long time to dry, even with a dryer.

—If your hair is seriously damaged or if your scalp is irritated. (Your stylist will be able to advise you in choosing which products to use and how often you should wash your hair.)

ABOUT YOUR BRUSH AND COMB . . .

Don't forget to wash your brushes and combs, including the ones in your purse and in your desk at work. If you don't, you'll only be brushing and combing dirt and oils back into your shimmering clean hair. Los Angeles–based hair and beauty expert Riquette Hofstein admonishes her clients with, "If you don't, it's like taking a bath and then putting your dirty underwear back on."

THE HEAT IS ON

Before taking a sauna or steam bath, apply conditioner to your hair—concentrating on the ends—and cover with a plastic shower cap and a damp towel. The heat will help the conditioning oils and emollients penetrate the hair shaft.

Simply squirt a tiny bit of shampoo into both brush and comb and toss them into the sink whenever you wash your hair (or at least every other time). Comb loose hair from your brush and then rinse completely.

They will be dry again by the time you've finished styling your hair.

HELP YOUR NAILS

Protect your nails—as well as your hair and scalp—by wearing rubber kitchen gloves when washing your hair. You might even make your hair washing a part of your personal manicure. Lightly massage a dab of olive or corn oil into your cuticles before slipping your hands into the gloves. The heat of the water will warm the oil and soften your cuticles, making it easy to push them back.

7 BLOW-DRYING, ROLLING, AND OTHER STYLING BASICS

Has anyone actually *slept* on rollers since hot rollers and modern-day curling irons hit the market? We may have had occasion to use rollers, but they certainly aren't the bristle-and-wire rollers that interrupted our sleep patterns in the '60s and early '70s. Thankfully, today's cutting and styling techniques have put an end to that misery.

As long as you have a good haircut, you can do just about anything to your hair and it will look fine. It'll look sensational if you use the right styling products and techniques.

The more you work *with* your hair—acknowledging its type and texture—the easier your hairstyling regimen will be. Put another way: If your hair is naturally curly, don't expect to have a stick-straight style unless you're prepared to spend at least half an hour in front of your mirror juggling your dryer and a handful of styling goo.

THE RIGHT STUFF

If you're mousse-shy, recalling the early incarnations of scented foams and sprays designed to give hair body and make it hold a curl or wave, let me allay your fears. Today's styling aids are formulated to make your hair look beautiful and feel great, not stiff and sticky.

I have a friend who resisted using anything but shampoo and an occasional hot oil conditioning treatment for her thick but fine, straight hair. She was very limited in the styles she could wear—basically, it had to be a blunt bob, with or without bangs—because of her absolute refusal to use gels and mousse. "Those things make my hair a dirt magnet," she complained.

Then, while having her hair styled for her sister's wedding, she surrendered and allowed the stylist to use a bit of light styling gel before blowing her hair dry. "I was amazed! I figured I would have to jump into the shower as soon as I came home from the reception," she relates. "I had this full head of hair that looked really pretty. Even after I'd danced all night at the reception, it still looked—and felt—clean and full."

We can't dwell on our past experiences with perms and other products. The beauty business changes almost before our very eyes. The industry is also extremely responsive to the needs of the consumer, sometimes creating products on the basis of customers' suggestions or requests.

Let's take a guided tour of today's hairstyling marketplace:

- *Styling gel*, also known as *setting gel* or just plain *gel:* Probably the most versatile styling product you'll use, gel comes in varying degrees of holding power.

    Liquid or gel sprays merely add body and volume to hair, while stronger products offer medium to firm control. Just remember that, if you're in a hurry, reach for the liquid or spray versions. Regular gels, even those offering light control, take a long time to dry.

- *Forming gel,* also known as *sculpting gel:* Descended from the Brilliantine and cream hair tonics Grandpa used, these products allow you to actually shape your hair into waves or curls that won't budge once hair is dry and clips are removed. These products are perfect for wet-look styles, since hair has that shiny finish even when it's dry.
- *Mousse,* or *styling cream* or *foam:* The consistency of meringue, these lightweight products are usually packaged in pressurized containers. They add lift and body to hair, especially when applied to the roots. The main drawback to these products is that, if you use too much, hair gets dusty-looking once dry.
- *Heat-activated styling spray:* The newest body-builders on the market, these products react to heat, either from hot rollers, steam rollers, curling irons, or blow dryers. Rather like ordinary hair spray, they come in aerosol and non-aerosol varieties. Lotion and spray gels are also available.

Other styling products you might find useful are silicon sprays that add sheen to your hair and give it that patent leather or wet look; sealing lotions and sprays that flatten the hair's cuticle and restore that delicate two percent acid mantle to your hair and scalp; styling sprays and conditioning sprays with sunscreen to hold your style while protecting your hair from environmental damage.

Before you rush out and buy everything on the shelf, ask your hairdresser to recommend what you need for your own hair type and style. Also be aware that the most expensive product may not be the best product for your hair. Some of those "vitamin" and "natural" additives may jack up the price of the product while doing very little for your hair and scalp. Hair is ninety-seven percent protein and nothing in the world—except another protein—can actually fuse with the medulla to repair damage or alter the condition of your hair.

GET SET

If you are out of styling gel, comb witch hazel or stale beer through damp hair. For more hold, use a tablespoon of sugar dissolved in a cup of warm water.

ADDED "AMMO"

You will also want to have many of these items in your beauty arsenal:

—A comb with wide, rounded teeth for gentle styling.
—A hair pick to lift and fluff curly hair.
—A rat-tail comb to lift and shape your hair.
—An assortment of brushes, from round natural-bristle styling brushes in various sizes to a curved, vented brush with round-tipped plastic bristles.
—A handful of long metal hair clips to hold waves in place.
—Two handfuls of small metal hair clips or plastic-tipped bobby pins for pin curls.
—Plastic-tipped hairpins for chignons, French rolls, and other special upswept hairdos.
—Assorted covered elastic bands, headbands, barrettes, and combs.

—A pistol-grip blow dryer, with diffuser and directional funnel attachments.

—A set of electric curlers, preferably with velour-covered rollers, or soft, spongy steam rollers.

—End papers, if you use Velcro or bristled rollers or if your hot rollers have little spikes all over them.

—A curling iron (preferably with a heat control and/or steam features) for touch-ups. You might want to have several sizes to make a variety of curls.

—A hand mirror that's large enough to give you a look at the back of your head . . . or, better yet, a large mirror attached to the wall opposite your bathroom or vanity mirror. This allows you a full view—front, back, and sides!

Once you have assembled your styling products and tools, you're ready to style your hair.

WHAT A WAY TO BLOW!

The hand-held hair dryer is without a doubt the most important styling aid of the twentieth century. Used correctly, it can make curly hair straight, shape straight hair into soft curls, fluff any length hair into loosely shaped lines.

The basic technique is simple:

Step 1: After washing hair and combing out any tangles with a wide-tooth comb, apply styling gel, volumizing spray, or styling product of your choice and comb through hair.

Step 2: Using your comb, part your hair, first in the center, across the top and back to the nape, then horizontally, across the back. This enables you to work with a small area at a time.

Step 3: Starting at the bottom, lift hair—either with a comb, vented brush, or round styling brush, or even with your fingertips—and direct air toward the roots. *Use only medium to low temperatures to avoid damaging your hair.*

Step 4: Work your way to the crown, moving and shaping hair as desired. Let each section cool before releasing hair from brush or you will lose what you've just worked for.

Step 5: Finish with a light spritz of hair spray.

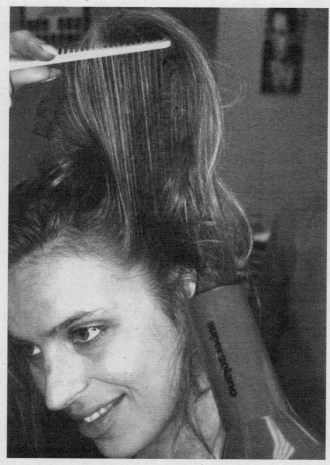

Blow volume into long, straight hair and create rolling waves about the face for a sexy, sophisticated evening look. Work a little styling gel into wet hair, concentrating on the roots but combing it lightly to the ends. Lift hair in sections with a brush

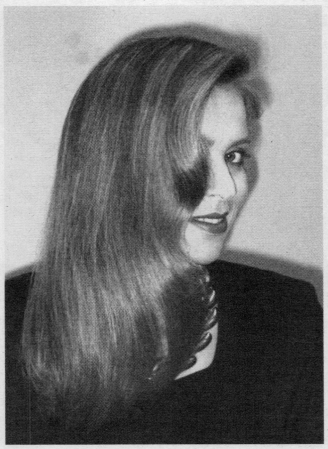

or comb. Concentrate the air flow at the roots, then work to the ends. When hair is almost dry, make a straight part high on one side. Then lift each section with a curved brush and move into place, shaping a sweeping wave over one brow and rolling ends under. A spritz of hair spray will hold everything in place.

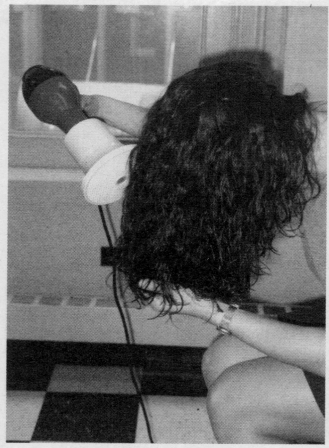

Lightly layered to distribute its weight, and blunt cut at the base, this versatile cut has lots of styling possibilities. With the diffuser attachment to soften the dryer's air flow and a bit of styling gel to enhance the wave of the hair, just lean over, flip your hair over your head, and dry away. Scrunch hair with

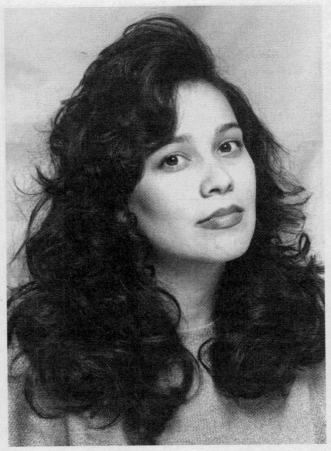

your fingers, then, when almost dry, toss hair back. Use your fingertips and a vented brush to finish styling. Distribute loosely about your shoulders for this casual style. Diffusing is a great way to style hair with a moderate amount of natural curl or a gentle body wave.

REVITALIZE DARK HAIR

Give dark hair a lift with weekly conditioning treatments you can make at home. Steep 3 tablespoons dried rosemary in 1 cup milk overnight in a covered jar (in the fridge, of course). When ready to use, strain liquid to remove rosemary. To this liquid, stir in 1 egg and 1 tablespoon honey. Massage this mixture into your hair and cover with plastic wrap for 30 minutes before shampooing.

LOOK AT THOSE CURLS!

Don't think the art of pin curls has been blown away by the hand-held dryer. This is a sensational way to create lively curl . . . especially in short, layered hair.

Step 1: Comb styling lotion through damp hair.

Step 2: Part hair into sections, according to the design of your style. The smaller the section the tighter the curl.

Step 3: Twist hair around your index finger and lay curl against your scalp. Secure with a clip or plastic-tipped bobby pins.

To make stand-up pin curls, twist hair and form an upright loop rather than placing hair flat against the head. Insert clip through the loop and secure ends at the scalp.

Step 4: Dry hair completely, using either a hooded dryer or a pistol-grip blow dryer with diffuser attachment.

Step 5: Let hair cool before removing clips.

Step 6: Brush gently into place. Complete styling by lifting hair with a pick or your fingertips.

In case you're curious, the difference between traditional, flat pin curls and the stand-up kind is that flat curls are usually tighter; stand-up curls are livelier and looser.

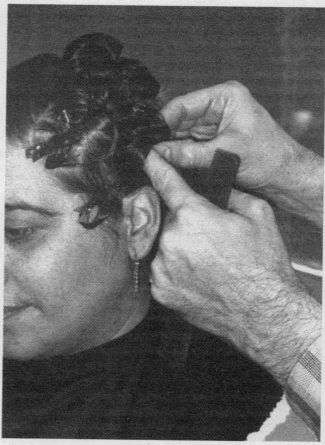

A great way to give short, fine hair body and curl is to cut it in layers, then treat it to a soft body wave. Give the curl a lift by setting gelled hair in flat pin curls around the face and nape. Make stand-up curls across the crown and back. Dry with diffused air and let cool completely before removing clips. Brush

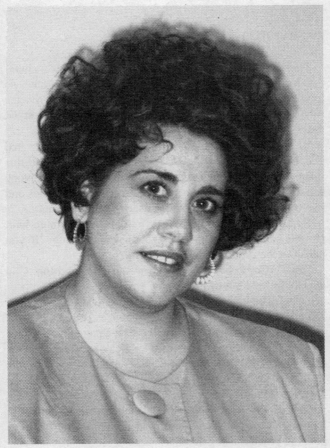

gently upward with a vented brush. Comb waves across the forehead; clip into place and spray for hold. Loosen curls through the crown and across the back; brush upward with your fingertips. A bit of hair spray will secure curl. Remove clips and you have a dynamic day-to-night look.

BRUSH UP ON CURL

There's one problem with blow-dry styling: It's sometimes difficult to make hair hold its style because it takes so long to roll your hair around brushes and blow it dry. By the time you've finished drying and are ready to finish the style, those first curls you made have lost their bounce.

Richard Peterson, a talented stylist who coifs celebrated clients at New York's famed Kenneth's Salon, devised this imaginative technique for lasting wave and curl that anyone can do. You will need two or three large round brushes and two or three medium or small brushes for this method.

Step 1: Comb your chosen styling product through hair, parting hair as you normally would when styling. (If you part it in the middle, make that part.)

Step 2: Comb hair forward from the sides and top. Clip loosely to hold out of the way as you work.

Step 3: Beginning at the bottom in back, section hair and roll around medium or large round brushes.

NOTE: Rolling hair under will create a pageboy look; upward makes a flip. If you form vertical—up and down—rolls, you will create lush waves as you finish your style. Roll hair toward your face for a gentle frame; back for graceful fullness.

Step 4: After you roll and dry each curl, leave brush in hair and pick up the section of hair above that curl and repeat the process using another brush.

Step 5: As each curl cools, remove that brush and use it for another curl.

Step 6: Roll hair in front, using brushes in varying sizes to add texture to the curls that will frame your face.

Step 7: Finish your style by gently brushing hair into place. Add spray for light hold.

THE RUDIMENTS OF ROLLING

Regardless of the type of rollers you use, the technique is still the same:

Step 1: Comb styling product through hair.

Step 2: Starting at the center on top, part hair in sections as wide as the roller you plan to use. The direction of your part is determined by your style. Hair rolled parallel with your hair line in either direction will look one way; vertical, or up-and-down, rolls will look another.

Step 3: Pick up a section of hair, one-half to one inch thick, and comb straight up. Wrap end with paper if desired. *Always* use end papers if your hair is damaged or if you use brush or Velcro rollers or spiked hot rollers.

Step 4: Position roller at end of hair and, without pulling or applying tension to roots, roll hair under.

Step 5: Secure with a clip close to the head. Take care that you don't bend hair back at the root.

Step 6: Dry naturally or under hooded dryer.

Step 7: Cool completely, then remove clips and rollers.

Step 8: Brush hair gently to remove impressions made by rollers.

Step 9: Style as desired.

Step 10: Spray lightly for lasting hold.

To vary the degree and direction of your curls, use an assortment of curlers—small, medium, and large—rolled in random directions. Just take care that you don't pull or put pressure on the roots of your hair.

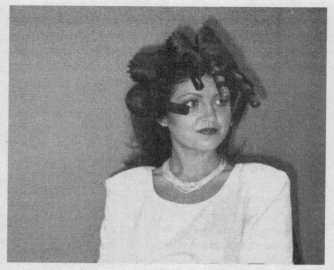

Hair is cut in layers to distribute its volume beautifully about the face. Apply strong-holding gel at the roots, then comb to distribute gel lightly through to the ends. Section hair, combing sides and top forward. Clip extra hair to hold loosely out of the way. Then, starting at the bottom in back, lift hair in sections and roll around medium or large round brushes. As each curl is blown dry and rolled, leave brush in hair and pick up the section of hair above that curl and repeat the process. As curls cool, remove brushes. Roll hair in front, using brushes in varying sizes to graduate curl. Finish your style by gently brushing hair into place. Back comb lightly through the crown for height. Add spray for light hold.

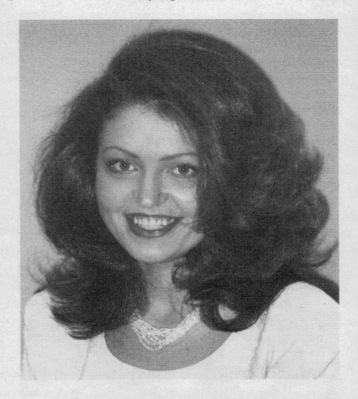

If you are using electric rollers or steam rollers, heat according to the manufacturer's instructions. You may find it helpful to use a styling lotion or spray formulated for heat styling.

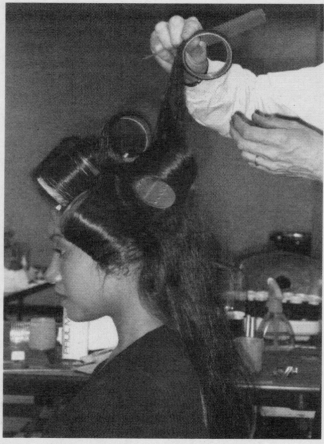

Lush and sophisticated, this is a stunning rich girl look, perfect for long, thick locks. With super-holding styling gel combed from the roots to the ends, roll hair away from your face on jumbo curlers. If unrolled hair dries before you have set it, spritz it with a little water. Using either a hooded dryer or a

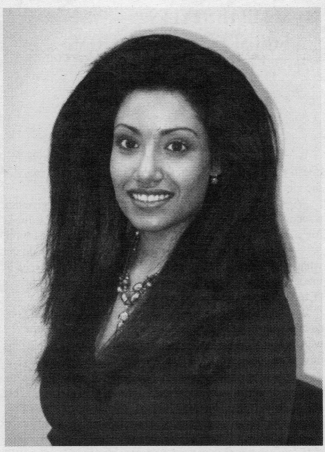

pistol-grip dryer with diffuser attachment, dry hair completely.
Let cool before removing curlers. Lift hair in sections and
back-comb gently through the crown and at the sides to create
fullness. Smooth hair into place for a smooth silhouette.

8 SPECIAL STYLES FOR SPECIAL SITUATIONS

We all have those times when our regular hairstyle just doesn't work, when a quickie blow-dry or simple twirl of the electric rollers or curling iron just isn't enough.

Wigs and hairpieces might do the trick, but don't give this a second thought unless you're ready to fork over the funds for a top quality product. This is *not* a place to scrimp. Where wigs and hairpieces are concerned, you really do get what you pay for. While there are some dazzling pieces at moderate prices, most low-priced fake hair fairly shrieks "Cheap!"

If you do decide to buy a hairpiece, look for a high concentration of hair strands woven into a well-constructed weft. (That's the heavy mesh that you slip the hairpins through to hold your spare hair to your head.)

Today's synthetic fibers are every bit as natural-looking as their human hair counterparts, though real hair wigs *feel* more lifelike. Also, natural hair wigs can be styled more easily than their man-made counterparts which are constructed to look a certain way and stay that way, come rain or shine.

If you take proper care of both hair and wig base, you'll have plenty of styling options to choose from for a year or more.

If you've ever wondered what you'd look like with red or

blond hair or with a style very different from what you're accustomed to, just pay a visit to a wig shop and have a ball!

If you're serious about adding wigs, falls, and pieces to your hairstyling bag of tricks, consult your haircare professional to direct you to a reliable source of wig products. And ask him or her to teach you how to take care of them properly.

Weaves and extensions are not for the woman of little commitment. While a wig or piece can be popped on or off in minutes, the weaving process is both time-consuming and costly. It involves entwining small clusters of hair—usually curls or tiny braids—into small sections of the hair growing from the head. (Although it *can* be done on straight hair, this styling technique really doesn't work well on straight hair.)

I won't even discuss the extensions that are applied with an adhesive that's akin to the hot glue we all have used for arts and crafts projects aside from saying don't do it. This process can do serious damage to your hair.

Hair weaving takes *ten to twelve hours* for a full head of hair. Done properly, it lasts about six weeks with proper care and intermittent tightening of those tiny knots. (Tightening can take as long as four hours.) Still, done well, the results of a weave can be outstanding.

Woven or braided hairstyles can be washed—after all, you still need to clean your scalp—but this must be done with care. Use just a tiny bit of shampoo. Rub your hands together and massage gently into your scalp. Then rinse, using plenty of tepid water, until it runs clear. Pat the excess water from your hair and then let it dry. Don't do this every day or you'll shorten the life of your weave.

EXTEND YOUR STYLE

When I visited the New York campus of the Learning Institute of Beauty Sciences I spotted one of the best-looking weaves I'd seen in a long time. Student Jacqueline Burke had added a shoulder-length cascade of curl to the shorter, thinner hair of her classmate Ann Castillo.

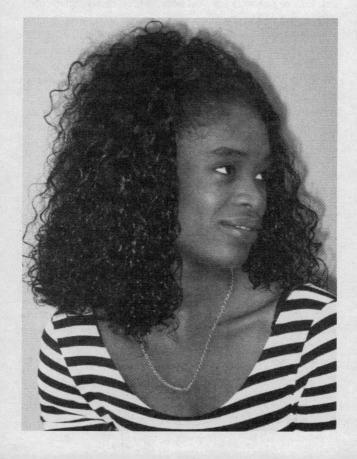

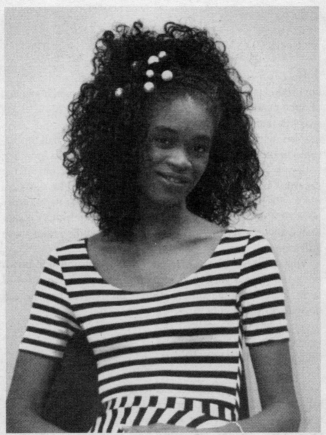

Jacqueline coiled Ann's hair to her head and worked the extensions from the crown. The only "real" hair you see in these pictures is the waved section in front on top. The results were stunning. A bit of decoration is added to the top with a cluster of pearl-topped hairpins in assorted sizes tucked among the waves and curls.

ACCESSORIES AND ASSORTED TRICKS

Hair accessories like barrettes, combs, headbands, fabric-covered elastic circles that look like flowers when twisted about a handful of hair, even extensions and scarves are easy ways to tame a wild mane.

Well, what do *you* do when that great guy you met this afternoon on the beach calls at 6:30 to invite you to tonight's sold-out 8 o'clock concert . . . and you just got out of the shower? I, for one, reach for my gel and barrette with the black silk bow and slick everything back to the nape of my neck. It's not particularly original, but it's definitely faster than blow-dry styling and infinitely more stylish than loose and stringy.

You can also create elegant French rolls, upside-down pony tails and a variety of braids to give your hair a lot of style. Here are some simple styling alternatives anyone can do with a little practice.

DRESS UP YOUR HAIR IN MINUTES

Actress Lynette Sheldon has long, fine hair that she usually wears loose about her shoulders. It is cut with bangs across the forehead and long layers that curve about her face. In hot weather, she pulls it back with a wide barrette or elastic band.

But what about special occasions? Richard Peterson, who has a long list of celebrity and society clients in New York, Palm Beach, and Cleveland, taught her how to create two dramatic, upswept looks without a rubber band.

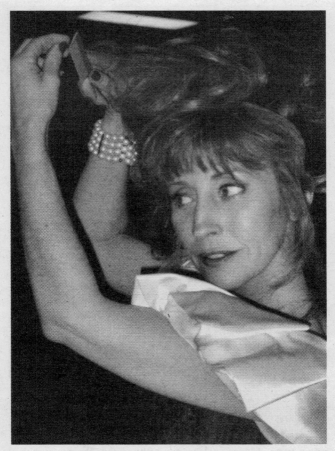

Lynette brushes her hair upward, like making a ponytail on top. She twists her hair two or three times, and secures it with hairpins at the crown. She lightly teases her hair and shapes it

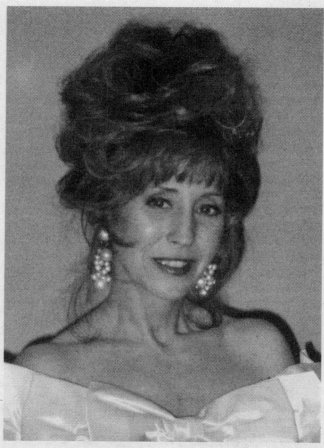

into a tiara of loose curls on top of her head. Wisps are pulled free at the sides and at the nape, and bangs are combed across the brow. A spritz of hair spray will hold this dazzling look in place as she dances the night away. The second, more sophisti-

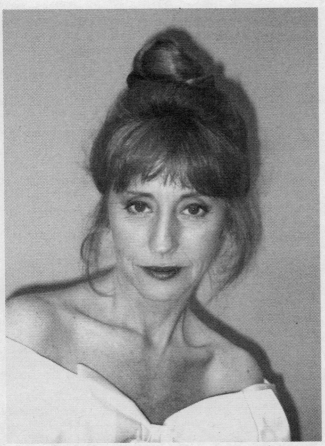

cated look, begins the same way; however, instead of teasing, hair is combed smooth and twisted into an asymmetrical knot at the crown. A hairpin or two will hold this great look in place.

PARLEZ VOUS FRENCH ROLL?

The French Roll, also called the French Twist, is one of the most elegant, classic hairstyles ever. Mid-length to long hair is combed smoothly to one side and then rolled back to the opposite direction and pinned into place. The result is sophisticated . . . simplicity at its most stunning, bringing to mind such movie beauties as Grace Kelly and Audrey Hepburn.

London Hair's Frances London DuBose has developed an innovative, foolproof way to make a French Roll with minimal effort. It's ideal for hair that is at least shoulder-length.

STEPS TO A SENSATIONAL FRENCH ROLL

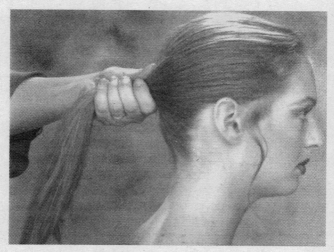

Step 1: **Comb hair off the face, gathering it into a ponytail.**

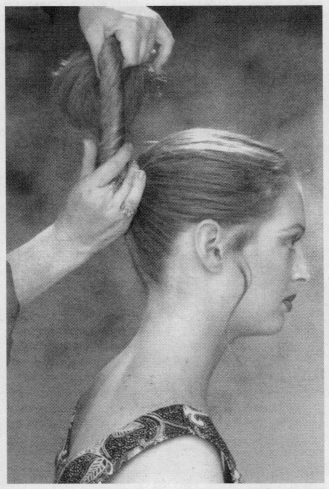

Step 2: Lift upward and begin twisting ponytail, holding taut at the back of the head.

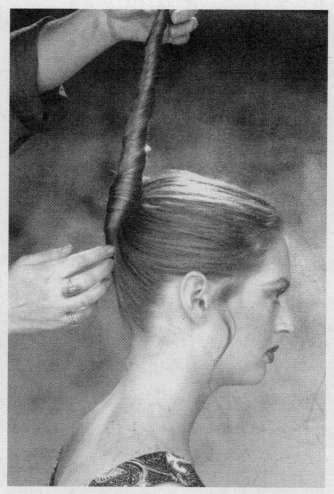

Step 3: Continue twisting until length of hair is coiled.

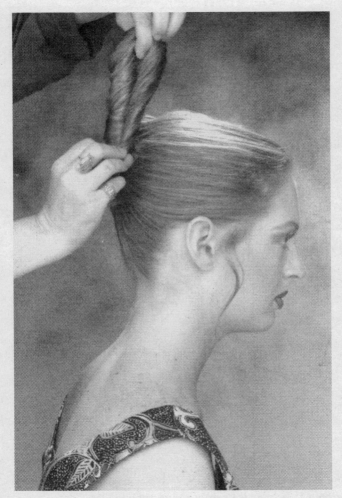

Step 4: Fold long end of hair over and tuck under. Secure tip with a hairpin if necessary.

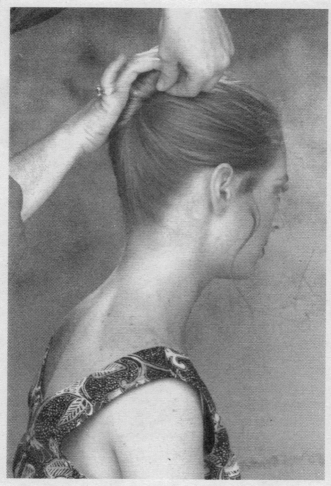

Step 5: Twist coiled hair over and pin into place.

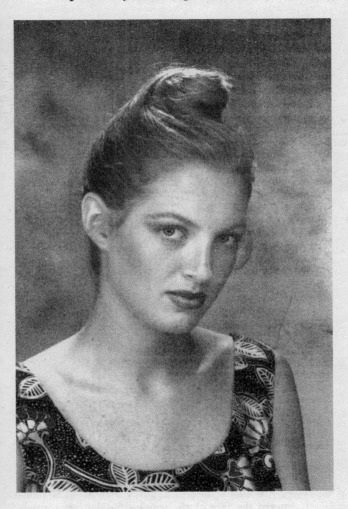

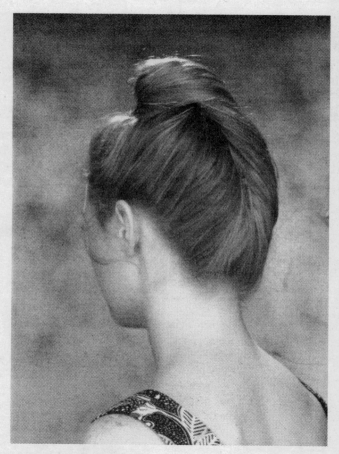

THE FINISHED TWIST
From every angle, this twist swirls gracefully up the back of the
head to a gentle knot at the crown. Wispy tendrils can be pulled
loosely toward the face at the temples for delicate softness.
HAIRSTYLE AND PHOTOS BY FRANCES LONDON DuBOSE.

NOT YOUR ORDINARY PONYTAIL

Anybody can pull their hair back and stick it through an elastic band and call it a Ponytail. It's a super-casual look, perfect for keeping your hair out of your face while you do the housework or go for a run. But what if you want a little style?

London Hair's Stephani McCrary has devised what she calls an Upside-down Ponytail. By inverting the length of the hair under the elastic, she creates a beautiful chevron at the nape. This is a simple process that requires absolutely no special equipment—just a comb—to produce results similar to those of a little plastic loop we've all seen on television.

You can also pull hair from the top and sides and make an Upside-down Ponytail at the back of the crown. Brush hair loosely about your shoulders for a slightly Alice-in-Wonderland look.

Or you can make two or three tails in a row from the crown, incorporating the ends of the top tail into the one below it for an intricate pattern.

Here's how to do it:

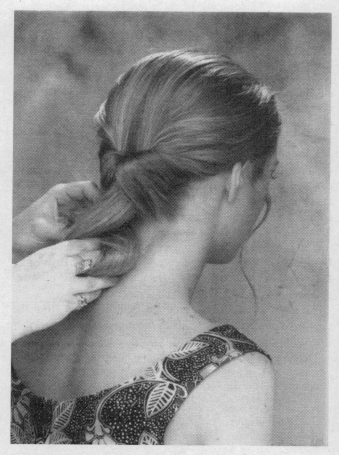

HOW TO MAKE AN UPSIDE-DOWN PONYTAIL

For an innovative Upside-down Ponytail, brush your hair to the back and catch it with a covered elastic band. Comb out any tangles and then gather the tail in one hand. Twist hair lightly to make it easier to handle. Lift the tail with one hand

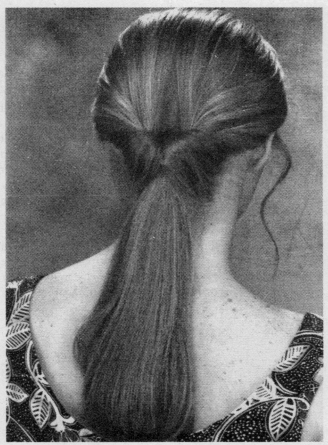

and insert it on top of the elastic band. Pull hair through, be-
hind the band, creating this smashing Upside-down Ponytail.
Comb ends of the tail so that hair falls beautifully down your
back. HAIRSTYLE BY STEPHANI McCRARY FOR LONDON
HAIR. PHOTO BY FRANCES LONDON DuBOSE.

THE BASICS OF BRAIDING

Those pigtails that took so long to make when we were in the first grade have come of age. These are grown-up plaits—French Braids and Fishtails or Herringbones—that can tame the wildest mane.

Hair need not be thick and long, though length helps. It doesn't even have to be all the same length. You can braid hair that is cut in long layers by incorporating it into your braid as you plait. Just part your hair into three or four sections and entwine them, one over the other, until you have braided your way from the crown or temples, as the case may be, to the nape.

As you can see, this is not something an ordinary person can do on her own head easily, but with practice it can be done. Initially, I suggest asking someone else to do this for you so you'll have the most beautiful braid possible.

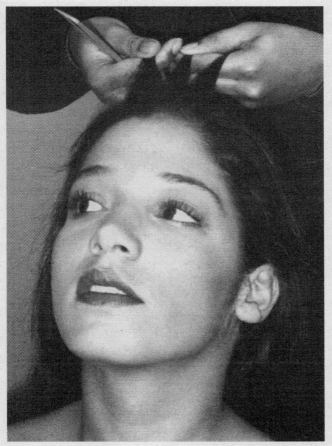

Start your braid by parting hair into three sections for a
French Braid, four for a Fishtail.

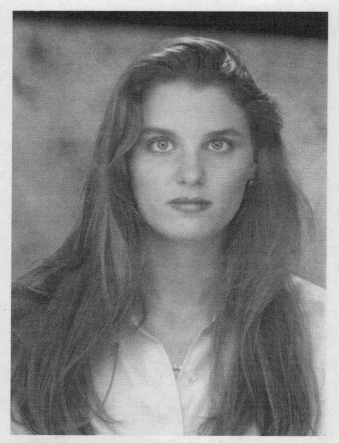

THE FRENCH CONNECTION

One of the most elegant braids we can make is the French Braid, which brings your hair off the face into a delicate rope down the center back of your head. Starting at your front hairline, part your hair into three sections from front to back. Begin the braid by lifting a section, about one inch thick, from

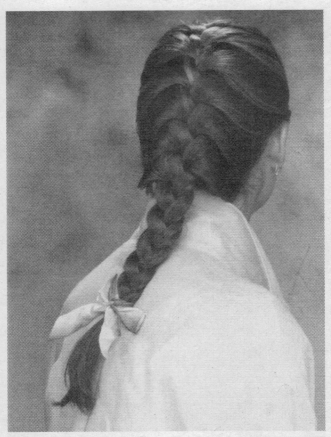

each and crossing the outside right section over the center section, placing it in the middle. Then lift and cross the outside left section over to the center into the middle. The original center piece is now in the bottom right position. Move this piece across the top right piece to the center. Keep working, left to the center, then right to the center, over the crown to the back of the

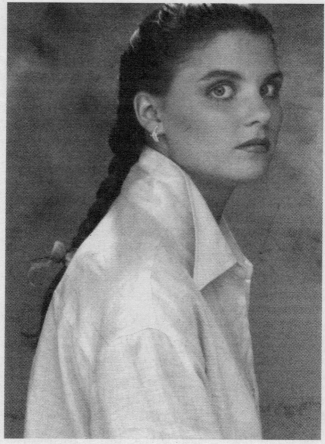

head. Pick up new hair from each section as you work your way down. When you have reached the nape, continue braiding until all hair is included in the plait. Tie off with a covered elastic band and add a pretty bow. HAIRSTYLE BY STEPHANI Mc-CRARY. PHOTOS BY FRANCES LONDON DuBOSE.

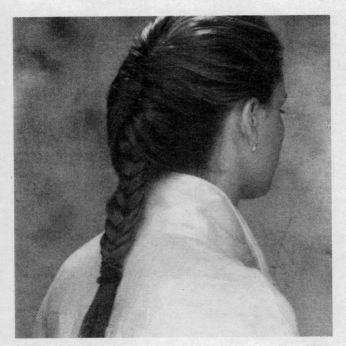

THE FISHTAIL BRAID

Here's a four-part approach to braiding you might want to try. For the Fishtail Braid, comb hair into four sections, front to back, which you will work one over two. The outside right part is placed over the middle two. Then the outside left is moved over the middle two. Take care to hold each section between your fingers to keep them separate. After four plaits, each section will have been moved to the outside and worked into the braid. This process is repeated until all hair is pulled into a stunning braid that starts just below the crown. When you reach the nape, continue working with all four sections, using all or some of the remaining length, to create a free-spirited Fishtail. Secure with a covered elastic band. HAIRSTYLE BY STEPHANI McCRARY. PHOTOS BY FRANCES LONDON DuBOSE.

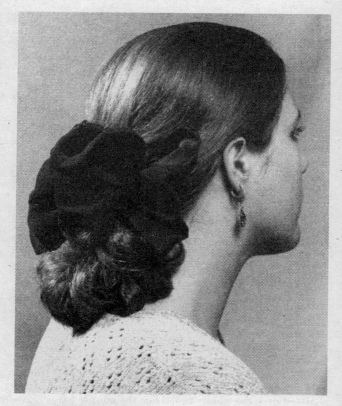

ELEGANT SIMPLICITY

Like that little black dress, a floppy black double bow made of silk chiffon attached to a big barrette is a fashion must. It will transform a casual mid-length or shoulder-length cut into a sophisticated, elegant evening look in minutes. Comb hair off the face and clip at the nape with the barrette. If you have bangs, fluff them softly across the forehead; otherwise slick hair back with gel for a smooth silhouette. PHOTO BY JORGE OCHOA.

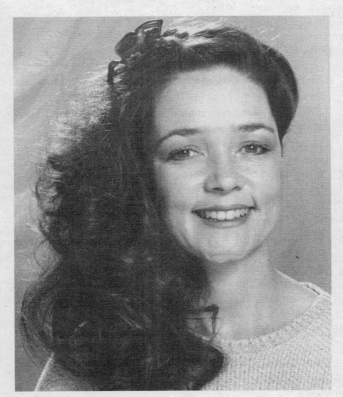

CLEVER CLIP

Singer Mary Foster Conklin has a lot of baby-fine hair that is lightly layered about the face. She needs a body wave to enhance movement as it cascades about her shoulders. Light styling gel guarantees volume, while steam rollers create lasting curl. For special occasions—such as performances in New York cabarets—Mary brushes her hair up and over to one side and secures it with a sassy butterfly clip. The back is smooth, with curls falling in a flurry across the shoulder. HAIRSTYLE BY COLIN LIVELY. PHOTO BY JORGE OCHOA.

MORE TREATS AND TRICKS . . .

- Make a narrow French braid across your head—from one temple to the other, about one inch back from the hairline. Brush remaining hair free, lifting from underneath to create volume. The result is a sophisticated headband.
- Create whimsical texture in your long, curly hairstyle by making tiny braids randomly throughout your hair—some using hair from the crown, others with hair from the under layers. Coil remaining hair around your curling iron to make vertical spirals. Shake your head to loosen the curls.
- Make French braids on each side of your head, working from the temples to the back and secure at the nape. Remaining hair can either be brushed into loose waves or incorporated into a single plait down your back.
- Keep tightly braided or cornrowed hair fresh looking by keeping your scalp clean. You can dab an alcohol-free astringent onto your scalp with a cottonball *or* you can cover your head with a stocking cap and gently wash your hair and scalp through the fabric. Finish by applying a light conditioning hair oil to the scalp. A cornrow style can last for weeks!

9 NEVER HAVE ANOTHER BAD HAIR DAY

At one time or another, everybody has trouble getting their hair to look the way they want it to. Straight hair lies flat against the head no matter how much lifting and curling it gets; curly hair remains untamed, looking more like a irate poodle than a stylish woman. It's a "bad hair day."

The cause could be something simple, such as ninety percent humidity that makes your hair frizz or, it might be that you're using the wrong styling products and it has you looking like you've plopped a string mop atop your head.

Or it could be more serious. Your hair may be damaged by the sun or winter's cold, dirt and dust in the air, chlorine from a swimming pool; by too many perms, applications of color or other chemical processes . . . or by hot rollers, curling irons, and blow drying.

Or your hair could be showing the ravages of ill health. Our hair is one of the first places our bodies show disease. Dull, brittle hair or hair that is excessively oily is an indicator that the body is out of whack in some way. It could be that you're fighting the flu or fending off an infection. Malnutrition, a diet high in fats and processed sugars and flours, as well as eating disorders, such as anorexia and bulimia, can show up as dramatic hair loss, drying, excessive oil, and breakage.

Stress also takes its toll on our hair, stripping hair of its sheen and even its color. Believe it or not, if you are ill or have been under serious stress, you may see that your hair has begun to turn gray. This is more apparent in lighter hair colors.

Our task is to pay attention to what our hair is telling us, following its condition on a day-to-day basis, and act accordingly. If not, we run the risk of serious damage and even permanent hair loss. Yes, women go bald too.

If you kill those follicles, you won't have any hair to grow.

NO DANDRUFF, NATURALLY

Put an end to flaky dandruff without expensive shampoos or medications. Once a week, massage oil of nettle or oil of rosemary into your scalp, then cover your head with a plastic shower cap or plastic wrap. Let stand for twenty minutes and wash with a gentle shampoo in warm water. For your final rinse, add 1 tablespoon dried fennel, nettles, or rosemary leaves to 2 cups boiling water, remove from heat, and steep until cool. Strain and pour through hair.

The only guaranteed way to get rid of split ends is to cut them off. You should be aware that some of the products that are marketed to *repair* splits only serve to further the problem. They contain waxes that adhere to the hair shaft and, since they build up, make it brittle. Then you're faced with a breakage problem.

We have to catch these conditions before we need a crew-cut. Strike up a partnership with your stylist to restore your hair and scalp to health and beauty. Find out what products you should be using . . . and how to use them. And make sure that you have regular trims, even if you're maintaining a length or if you want to grow it out.

MASSAGE MESSAGE

This tip gets to the root of year-round hair care: Gently massage your scalp with the tips of your fingers—or ask someone you love to do it—to stimulate blood circulation to each and every follicle. A healthy scalp leads to a healthy head of hair!

PAMPER YOUR HAIR

Keep your hair clean and in good condition and it will always look shiny and radiant. Even in wintertime, shampoo hair daily, using the mildest shampoo for your hair type. You want to remove soot and other airborne pollutants that get stuck to your hair and scalp.

Constant temperature changes—such as every time you step from that dry, overheated office building into the cold, or from air conditioning into the heat and humidity—can be treacherous to your tresses. Cover hair with a scarf or hat. This bit of shade makes you feel cooler in the summertime by keeping the top of your head from becoming too hot, and it slows the loss of body heat so you'll stay warmer when you're out of doors in the wintertime.

Another reminder: Keep your hatbands clean. Rub a bit of alcohol on a soft cloth around the inner band to remove sebaceous oil and dirt buildup. You don't want to mush that gunk into your freshly washed hair, do you?

COOL MOVE

I can't repeat it enough: A prevalent cause of hair damage is blow-drying at high temperatures. It can be devastating. Whenever possible, dry hair naturally. If you must blow hair dry, blot out most of the moisture with a thick, cotton terry towel and use a medium or low temperature setting as you brush or finger-comb hair into place. Avoid overdrying at all costs. This process may take a little longer, but it won't cremate your hair and scalp.

WATER WORKS ... AND SO DOES A GOOD DIET

Drink six to eight 8-ounce glasses of water—and we don't mean tea, coffee, or diet soda—every day, not only for your overall health but for the health of your hair and scalp.

With a little bit of know-how, the TLC of a good hairstylist, the right styling products, and a healthy diet, you truly will never have another bad hair day!

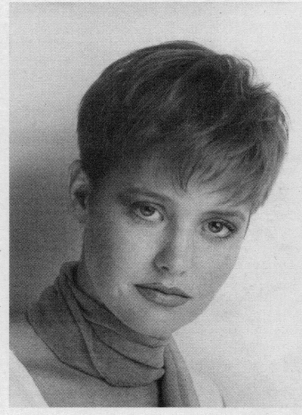

A great cut is key to having a healthy head of hair. This sophisticated short cut is ideal for baby-fine hair. Hair is cut very short to lie close to the head on the sides, curving easily over the ears, and tapering to the nape. Short layers on top fluff softly from the crown, providing a delicate frame for the face. A bit of styling gel will enhance the hair's lift. HAIRSTYLE AND PHOTO BY FRANCES LONDON DuBOSE.

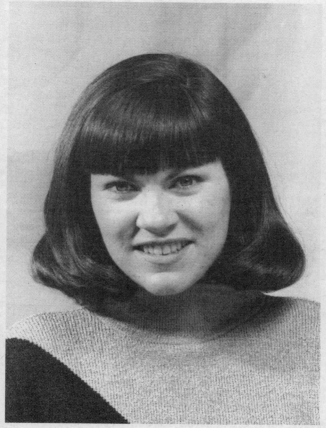

A stunning example of the beauty of healthy hair, this classic bob is blunt cut at the chin line, with long bangs that run straight across the brow line from temple to temple. Simply comb gel through damp hair and blow dry over a curved brush. Shape ends under to fashion a super-feminine pageboy. PHOTO BY JORGE OCHOA.

Naturally curly hair can be blown out into a straight style. For a sophisticated style, hair is gelled and shaped over a big, round brush. Robin Russo, herself a hairstylist, parts her thick, curly hair high on one side and then focuses the air flow of her dryer toward her hair, holding each section straight until it is completely dry. Whenever you use a hand-held dryer, make sure that you hold it at least seven inches from your hair . . . and *never* use it on high temperature.

ONE BASIC CUT . . .
A body worker and healer with a busy practice in New York City, Hattie Wiener needs a cut that will look good . . . no matter what. For this, her naturally curly hair is layered from the crown to distribute its weight gently about her face. Now in her late fifties, Hattie had dark hair as a girl. When she started turning gray, she began to color her hair. Once too monochromatic to be flattering, her hair now is natural-looking because of the low-lighting technique Colin Lively uses. He brushes mellow gold tones—from dark to light—throughout her hair, adding movement to the basic blond tone.

. . . TWO DYNAMIC STYLES
Hattie likes to start her day at full speed. This natural look needs absolutely no special attention. She simply finger-combs it into place and she's out the door!

For more formal occasions, Hattie can blow her hair out into a smoother, more sophisticated look. Hair is lifted with a vented brush and moved off the face from a soft side part. Hair curves slightly under to frame the face.

10 TWELVE TRICKS FOR TERRIFIC HAIR

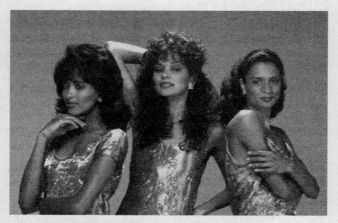

1 FABULOUS FAKERY

Create a great look—no matter how badly your own hair is be-having—by adding a wig or swatch of fantastic fake hair. A hairpiece is easy to wear and, if you follow directions, easy to care for. They won't damage your own hair either. Pictured, from left, are a softly curled wig with bangs that gently brush the brow; long, curly extensions applied with surgical glue, and a clip-on cluster of curls that cascade from the crown in dra-matic contrast to hair slicked back from the face with strong-hold styling gel. PHOTO COURTESY OF KANEKA AMERICA CORPORATION.

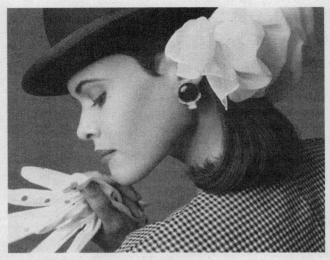

2 SOPHISTICATION IN A SNAP

Who hasn't gotten a last-minute invitation to lunch on a day when your hair looks absolutely awful? Here's a smart solution: Comb your short hair off your face and clip a swatch of fake hair at the nape. In this hairpiece, a large French clip barrette slips into a pocket in the webbing so that the hair falls from underneath a lush silk bow. If you like, top your new style with a sophisticated bowler and you're ready to go! No one will suspect your own hair is a mess. HAIRPIECE BY LOOK OF LOVE. PHOTO BY SUSAN JOHANN, COURTESY OF KANEKA AMERICA CORP.

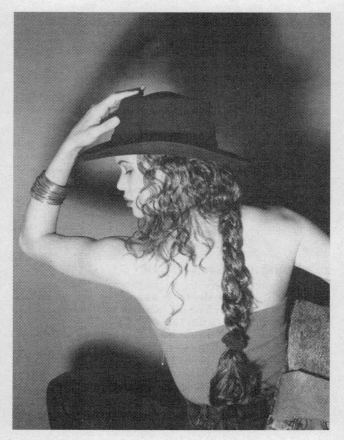

3 YEEHAW!

How's this for a fun way to salvage your hair? Just brave the wilds of fashion in a sassy cowboy hat. If that's not your style, you can go for a visored baseball hat, a straw sailor cap, or even a spangled evening cap. A hat may be a fashion accessory . . . but it can hide a multitude of problems!

4 A SPECIAL TWIST

Need a haircut and can't get to the salon? Just brush your hair back from your face, then lift a section of hair about one inch thick from one temple. Twist this hair into a simple coil that you direct to the back of your head. Clip it at the crown or, if you prefer, the center back. Repeat the process on the other side and secure both coils with a decorative barrette or bow. Comb remaining hair loosely about your shoulders. It's pretty and feminine, not to mention neat.

5 WRAP UP THAT PONYTAIL

Separate a section of hair from your ponytail and twist it around the elastic band. Secure it with a hairpin. This is a simple way to transform a classic ponytail into a remarkably grown-up style.

6 PERK UP!

You'll add bounce to any length hair if you scrunch waves into it. Blot out any excess water and spritz with spray gel, concentrating on the roots. Comb gently through the length of your hair. Then, starting at the roots, lift small sections of hair with your hand and squeeze it as you blow hair dry. Do your entire head and then finish with a soft spray. Run your fingers lightly through your hair for a loose, lazy curl.

7 RIBBONS AND BRAIDS

Add color to a long braid that runs down your back by working lengths of colorful ribbon through the sections of hair as you make the plait. Tie the tail off at the bottom with a matching bow.

8 CURLY CUES

Add clip-on curls to your everyday 'do to give it a sassy look. This little trick gives that tired, old, almost grown-out perm new life and adds shape to a sagging silhouette. You can select curls that match your natural color or go for fun, vibrant fashion colors that add highlights and contrast.

9 SECRET HAIR

Celebrity stylist Jose Eber has come up with an extraordinarily versatile way to add length, texture, and contrast to your hair with an exceptional product called Secret Hair. (You may have seen it on a late-night infomercial.) Lengths of hair are attached to interlocking combs, which hold the locks in place. This is a great way to add body to thinning hair and to dress up a sassy short cut.

10 MORE IS MORE

Pull your hair back into a thick ponytail at the crown and secure it with a colorful fabric-covered elastic. Then twist additional elastic bands at intervals down the length of your tail. You can do the same thing with bright and sparkly barrettes, too.

11 CREATIVE CASCADE

Lift shoulder-length hair back from your face and up from the nape. Grasp with one hand from underneath and twist it upward a couple of times and fasten it in the center back of your head with a large bow barrette. Let rest of hair fall loosely from the crown for a fresh, feminine style. This is another great styling trick for those occasions when you've been too long between haircuts!

12 CREATIVE COMBS

Comb hair back from the temples and hold it in place with a pair of combs or brush hair back and upward into a graceful twist that is held in place by a long, jewelled comb. Experiment with combs for a variety of beautiful, dress-up styles.

FOR YOU AND YOUR TODDLER

___ **GOOD-BYE DIAPERS** *Batya Swift Yasgur*
0-425-14185-3/$4.50

The parents' guide to successful, stress-free toilet training. *Good-bye Diapers* presents a variety of new techniques, enabling you to specifically design your child a complete toilet training program. Includes chapters on toilet training an older child, a one-day intensive program, and defining and preventing bedwetting.

___ **TIME-OUT FOR TODDLERS**
Dr. James W. Varni and Donna G. Corwin
0-425-12943-8/$8.00

This guide illustrates the revolutionary TIME-OUT method that benefits both child and parent, showing parents how to cope with common childhood behaviors—such as temper tantrums, sibling rivalry, whining, and selfishness—in a positive and effective manner.

___ **FOODS FOR HEALTHY KIDS**
Dr. Lendon Smith   0-425-09276-3/$4.99

Dr. Lendon Smith, America's leading authority on nutrition for children, tells how to prevent and alleviate health problems such as asthma, allergies, depression, constipation, hyperactivity, sleep problems and tension—not with medicine, but with good, nourishing food. He gives you his total nutrition program, complete with more than 100 recipes.